Telemedicine and Connected Health in Obstetrics and Gynecology

Editor

CURTIS LOWERY

OBSTETRICS AND GYNECOLOGY CLINICS OF NORTH AMERICA

www.obgyn.theclinics.com

Consulting Editor
WILLIAM F. RAYBURN

June 2020 • Volume 47 • Number 2

ELSEVIER

1600 John F. Kennedy Boulevard • Suite 1800 • Philadelphia, Pennsylvania, 19103-2899

http://www.theclinics.com

OBSTETRICS AND GYNECOLOGY CLINICS OF NORTH AMERICA Volume 47, Number 2
June 2020 ISSN 0889-8545, ISBN-13: 978-0-323-68384-5

Editor: Kerry Holland
Developmental Editor: Kristen Helm

Obstetrics and Gynecology Clinics (ISSN 0889-8545) is published quarterly by Elsevier Inc., 360 Park Avenue South, New York, NY 10010-1710. Months of issue are March, June, September, and December. Periodicals postage paid at New York, NY, and additional mailing offices. Subscription price per year is $325.00 (US individuals), $719.00 (US institutions), $100.00 (US students), $404.00 (Canadian individuals), $908.00 (Canadian institutions), $100.00 (Canadian students), $459.00 (international individuals), $908.00 (international institutions), and $225.00 (international students). To receive student/resident rate, orders must be accompanied by name of affiliated institution, date of term, and the signature of program/residency coordinator on institution letterhead. Orders will be billed at individual rate until proof of status is received. Foreign air speed delivery is included in all *Clinics* subscription prices. All prices are subject to change without notice. POSTMASTER: Send address changes to *Obstetrics and Gynecology Clinics*, Elsevier Health Sciences Division, Subscription Customer Service, 3251 Riverport Lane, Maryland Heights, MO 63043. **Customer Service: Telephone: 1-800-654-2452 (U.S. and Canada); 314-447-8871 (outside U.S. and Canada). Fax: 314-447-8029. E-mail: journalscustomerservice-usa@elsevier.com (for print support); journalsonlinesupport-usa@elsevier. com (for online support).**

Reprints. For copies of 100 or more of articles in this publication, please contact the Commercial Reprints Department, Elsevier Inc., 360 Park Avenue South, New York, New York 10010-1710. Tel.: 212-633-3874; Fax: 212-633-3820; E-mail: reprints@elsevier.com.

Obstetrics and Gynecology Clinics of North America is also published in Spanish by McGraw-Hill Interamericana Editores S.A., P.O. Box 5-237, 06500, Mexico; in Portuguese by Reichmann and Affonso Editores, Rio de Janeiro, Brazil; and in Greek by Paschalidis Medical Publications, Athens, Greece.

Obstetrics and Gynecology Clinics of North America is covered in MEDLINE/PubMed (Index Medicus), Excerpta Medica, Current Concepts/Clinical Medicine, Science Citation Index, BIOSIS, CINAHL, and ISI/BIOMED.

Contributors

CONSULTING EDITOR

WILLIAM F. RAYBURN, MD, MBA
Associate Dean, Continuing Medical Education and Professional Development, Distinguished Professor and Emeritus Chair, Obstetrics and Gynecology, University of New Mexico School of Medicine, Albuquerque, New Mexico

EDITOR

CURTIS LOWERY, MD
Professor and MFM, Department of Obstetrics and Gynecology, Director, University of Arkansas for Medical Sciences, Institute of Digital Health and Innovation, Little Rock, Arkansas

AUTHORS

JESSICA L. BUTLER, MPH
Research Manager, The American College of Obstetricians and Gynecologists, Washington, DC

LAURA E. CARR, MD
Fellow in Neonatology, Division of Neonatology, Department of Pediatrics, University of Arkansas for Medical Sciences, Little Rock, Arkansas

NATHANIEL DᴇNICOLA, MD, MSHP
The George Washington University School of Medicine & Health Sciences, The American College of Obstetricians and Gynecologists Taskforce on Telehealth, Washington, DC

STANLEY K. ELLIS, EdD
Assistant Professor, Director of Education, University of Arkansas for Medical Sciences, Institute for Digital Health and Innovation, Little Rock, Arkansas

DANIEL GROSSMAN, MD
Department of Obstetrics, Gynecology and Reproductive Sciences, Professor, Advancing New Standards in Reproductive Health (ANSIRH), Bixby Center for Global Reproductive Health, University of California, San Francisco, Oakland, California

RICHARD W. HALL, MD
Professor, Neonatology, Division of Neonatology, Department of Pediatrics, University of Arkansas for Medical Sciences, Little Rock, Arkansas

WILBUR C. HITT, MD, FACOG, FACOEM
Associate Professor, Department of Obstetrics and Gynecology, Florida International University, Miami, Florida

SIWON LEE, MD, PhD
Resident, Department of Obstetrics and Gynecology, Mount Sinai Medical Center, Miami Beach, Florida

CURTIS LOWERY, MD
Professor and MFM, Department of Obstetrics and Gynecology, Director, University of Arkansas for Medical Sciences, Institute of Digital Health and Innovation, Little Rock, Arkansas

EVERETT F. MAGANN, MD
Professor, Department of Obstetrics and Gynecology, MFM Division, Little Rock, Arkansas

KATHRYN MARKO, MD
Department of Obstetrics and Gynecology, The George Washington University School of Medicine & Health Sciences, The American College of Obstetricians and Gynecologists Taskforce on Telehealth, Washington, DC

JANET L. McCAULEY, MD, MHA, CPC, FACOG
Senior Medical Director, Blue Cross Blue Shield of North Carolina, Assistant Consulting Professor, Department of Obstetrics and Gynecology, Duke University School of Medicine, Durham, North Carolina

FRANSCESCA MIQUEL-VERGES, MD
Associate Professor, Division of Neonatology, Department of Pediatrics, University of Arkansas for Medical Sciences, Little Rock, Arkansas

CATHERINE J. MOORE, BS
Section on Gynecologic Oncology, Department of Obstetrics and Gynecology, Wake Forest School of Medicine, Winston-Salem, North Carolina

CLARE NESMITH, MD
Assistant Professor, Division of Neonatology, Department of Pediatrics, University of Arkansas for Medical Sciences, Little Rock, Arkansas

ABIGAIL M. RAMSEYER, DO
MFM Fellow, University of Arkansas for Medical Sciences, Little Rock, Arkansas

DAVID I. SHALOWITZ, MD, MSHP
Section on Gynecologic Oncology, Department of Obstetrics and Gynecology, Wake Forest University School of Medicine, Department of Implementation Sciences, Wake Forest School of Medicine, Winston-Salem, North Carolina

BARBARA L. SMITH, RN, BSN, UAMS
High-Risk Pregnancy Program, Guidelines Director, University of Arkansas for Medical Sciences, Little Rock, Arkansas

SARITA SONALKAR, MD, MPH
Assistant Professor, Department of Obstetrics and Gynecology, University of Pennsylvania, Philadelphia, Pennsylvania

LINDSEY B. SWARD, MD
Assistant Professor, Medical Student Clerkship Director, Department of Obstetrics and Gynecology, University of Arkansas for Medical Sciences, Little Rock, Arkansas

ANTHONY E. SWARTZ, BS, RT(R), RDMS
Director of Telemedicine Market Development, Education and Innovation, Department of Obstetrics and Gynecology, Duke University School of Medicine, Durham, North Carolina

CHAD B. TAYLOR, MD
Assistant Professor, University of Arkansas for Medical Sciences, Little Rock, Arkansas

TERRI-ANN THOMPSON, PhD
Senior Associate, Ibis Reproductive Health, Cambridge, Massachusetts

TARA VENABLE, MD
Assistant Professor, Division of Neonatology, Department of Pediatrics, University of Arkansas for Medical Sciences, Little Rock, Arkansas

JULIE R. WHITTINGTON, MD
MFM Fellow, University of Arkansas for Medical Sciences, Little Rock, Arkansas

ALEXANDRA WISE-EHLERS, MD
Resident Physician, University of Arkansas for Medical Sciences, College of Medicine, Little Rock, Arkansas

LINDA L.M. WORLEY, MD
Regional Associate Dean, Northwest Arkansas Campus, University of Arkansas for Medical Sciences (UAMS), College of Medicine, Professor of Psychiatry and Obstetrics and Gynecology, UAMS, Fayetteville, Arkansas; Adjunct Professor of Medicine, Vanderbilt, Nashville, Tennessee

Contents

> Digital health technologies improve outcomes within many health care fields. They include telemedicine and telehealth, remote patient monitoring, mobile health applications, data analytics, and social networking. Patients, providers, and insurers benefit from digital health, with time and cost savings as well as access to aggregate data, used to predict disease and outcomes and allowing tailored solutions. Some essentials of digital health implementation include champion providers, patients in need, technology, peer support system, understanding laws and regulations, seed funding, and sustainability. Successful programs can and will be established, leading health care into a more value-based future largely focused on direct-to-consumer care.

> Complexity in regulation and reimbursement of telehealth across the United States yields inconsistent use and availability of services. Drivers of this variation stem from existing regulatory, licensing, and payment policy that was designed for face-to-face care. Emerging technology for connected care continues to outpace the rules that govern its use. This article explores the drivers of uncertainty around regulation and payment of remote care services, and provides a roadmap for fulfillment of the benefits of connected care.

> Telemedicine has been used to expand access to routine prenatal care for patients in rural areas and areas without enough obstetrician/gynecologists. Telemedicine can be used to reduce face-to-face visits, to increase patient autonomy and satisfaction, for behavioral modification, and to aid in smoking cessation. Patients and providers alike find telemedicine a useful adjunct to routine care.

> Telemedicine involves the use of technology to provide services to patients and share medical information. Telemedicine's use has increased

as technology has advanced. It allows for medicine to be practiced from a distance to reach patients in rural or underserved areas. Telemedicine has widespread uses in high-risk obstetrics, including management of diabetes, diagnosis and management of hypertensive disorders of pregnancy, screening for fetal malformations with teleultrasound, delivering care to underserved areas, and more. The use of telemedicine to provide care to patients and information to health care providers at a distance has been well accepted by the patients and providers.

Telemedicine and telehealth (TM/TH) are the 2 terms used interchangeably focusing on the delivery of health care services at a long distance using telecommunication technology. TM/TH has several gynecologic applications, including the well-woman visits, preventive care, preconception counseling, family planning including contraception and medical abortion, infertility workup, teleradiology, cervical cancer screening and colposcopy, mental health, and telesurgery. The goals of TM/TH are not only improving quality of health care in patients and building a virtual community of physicians but also increasing convenience, efficacy, and decreasing medical cost. In gynecology, TM/TH plays an important role, especially in well-woman care.

Patients with gynecologic cancers experience better outcomes when treated by specialists and institutions with experience in their diseases. Unfortunately, high-volume centers tend to be located in densely populated regions, leaving many women with geographic barriers to care. Remote management through telemedicine offers the possibility of decreasing these disparities by extending the reach of specialty expertise and minimizing travel burdens. Telemedicine can assist in diagnosis, treatment planning, preoperative and postoperative follow-up, administration of chemotherapy, provision of palliative care, and surveillance. Telemedical infrastructure requires careful consideration of the needs of relevant stakeholders including patients, caregivers, referring clinicians, specialists, and health system administrators.

Telemedicine has the potential to increase access to family planning. The most common application involved the use of text message reminders and mobile apps. Text messaging increased knowledge in a variety of settings, but had no effect on contraceptive uptake and use. Two randomized studies found that text messaging improved continuation of oral contraceptives and injectables. Telemedicine provision of medication abortion included both clinic-to-clinic and direct-to-patient models of care.

Telemedicine provision of medication abortion has been found to be equally safe and effective as in-person provision. Some measures of satisfaction are higher with telemedicine. Telemedicine may improve access to early abortion.

Tele-education is the use of communications technologies to distribute knowledge from one health care provider to another when distance separates providers. At the University of Arkansas for Medical Sciences, tele-education has been used for more than two decades to educate and support rural obstetrician/gynecologists throughout the state. Tele-education at University of Arkansas for Medical Sciences incorporates numerous interactive videoconferences and other digital portals and platforms. Continued provider education through tele-education increases access to quality care and evidenced-based practices for rural populations and is an effective strategy in the battle against health care disparities.

OBSTETRICS AND GYNECOLOGY CLINICS

SERIES OF RELATED INTEREST

Clinics in Perinatology
www.perinatology.theclinics.com
Pediatric Clinics of North America
www.pediatrics.theclinics.com

THE CLINICS ARE AVAILABLE ONLINE!
Access your subscription at:
www.theclinics.com

Foreword

The Role of Telemedicine in Improving Women's Health Care

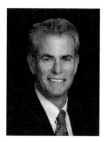

William F. Rayburn, MD, MBA
Consulting Editor

This issue of *Obstetrics and Gynecology Clinics of North America* focuses upon the important and timely subject of Telemedicine and Connected Health in Obstetrics and Gynecology. I was unable to uncover a text on this subject specifically for women's health providers, despite its remarkable relevance to health care delivery today. The University of Arkansas for Medical Sciences is known nationally for its statewide videoconferencing technologies to improve women's health care. The leader at Arkansas is Curtis Lowery, MD, who also serves as the very capable editor of this special issue.

Health care has been slow to transition to delivery systems that utilize remote technology, and it is encouraging that there are now many opportunities to use this technology to improve women's health care. Several articles in the issue discuss clinical applications of telemedicine in low-risk and high-risk obstetrics, gynecology, gynecologic oncology, and family planning. Compared with radiologists, psychiatrists, and emergency physicians, obstetricians and gynecologists have been among those specialists who use telemedicine the least to interact with patients. Telemedicine use is especially less common in smaller or physician-owned practices. The cost of implementation can be an impediment.

This text nicely answers the question, "What is the value of telemedicine?" It allows long-distance clinician and patient contact, care, advice, education, intervention, monitoring, and remote admissions. The American Telemedicine Association uses the terms telemedicine and telehealth interchangeably, although acknowledges that telehealth is sometimes used more broadly for remote health not involving direct clinical care. In contrast to telehealth that refers to a broader scope of remote health care services (especially distance learning), telemedicine relates to clinical services that are more individual patient based.

Telemedicine was originally created as a way to treat patients who lived in remote places. Rural and other underserved settings lack an ease of transportation, funding, or

Obstet Gynecol Clin N Am 47 (2020) xiii–xiv
https://doi.org/10.1016/j.ogc.2020.03.002
0889-8545/20/© 2020 Published by Elsevier Inc.

staff, and telemedicine may bridge the gap in access to care. Examples of telemedicine include physician-directed therapy done via digital monitoring instruments; tests being forwarded between facilities for interpretation by a specialist; home monitoring with continuous sending of patient health data; live client to practitioner online conferences; and even videophone interpretation of a consult during live procedures through remote access.

A similar health care delivery subject covered in this issue is connected health, a sociotechnical model for delivery using technology to provide services remotely. Connected health, also known as technology enabled care, aims to maximize health care resources and provide increased, flexible opportunities for consumers to engage with clinicians and better self-manage their care. It leverages readily available consumer technologies, such as mobile apps, to deliver patient care outside of the hospital or doctor's office.

A very relevant article in this issue pertains to regulation, licensing, and reimbursement in connected care. On average, a telemedicine visit costs much less than an office visit. Insurance claims filed for alternative settings of care have found that growth in telemedicine outpaced urgent care centers, retail clinics, and ambulatory surgical care centers. Telemedicine reduces unnecessary nonurgent emergency room visits, transportation expenses for regular checkups, and likely infant mortality when well implemented. It is used not only to replace face-to-face provider visits but also often to meet new demand. A primary disadvantage involves the continuing need for clearer, streamlined policies and standards using electronic health records about telemedicine and connected health. Professional liability seems to be low but needs more clarity.

Does health insurance cover telemedicine? There is no set standard for private health insurance providers regarding telemedicine. An in-person visit or real-time videochat between a physician and patient is often necessary for reimbursement. Some states have parity laws that require insurance companies to reimburse the same as in-person care for services provided. Most people have access to basic telecommunications technology, such as telephones, Internet, and computers. Improvements in computers and digital imaging, along with bandwidth availability and software, have made video conferencing an everyday event.

Dr Lowery's effort in editing this fine issue includes the broad experience of many authors who are well informed about their subjects. Information in these articles should prove to be helpful to our women's health care providers as they strive to implement optimal care to women within and outside their communities. Telemedicine technology can provide a compelling alternative to conventional acute, chronic, and preventive care, reduce cost, and improve clinical outcomes. The market is expected only to increase. I appreciate this overview and look forward to further developments in this promising option of health care delivery.

William F. Rayburn, MD, MBA
Department of Obstetrics and
Gynecology
University of New Mexico
School of Medicine
MSC 10 5580
1 University of New Mexico
Albuquerque, NM 87131-0001, USA

E-mail address:
wrayburn@salud.unm.edu

Preface

Intro to Telemedicine and Connected Health in Obstetrics and Gynecology

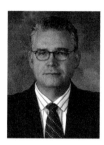

Curtis Lowery, MD
Editor

I would like to welcome you to this issue of *Obstetrics and Gynecology Clinics of North America* titled, "Telemedicine and Connected Health in Obstetrics and Gynecology." Health care costs have escalated over the last decade, and we have reached the point where we are spending nearly 20% of our gross national product on health care with little to show in quality for this expenditure. The justification for this spending relied on the superiority of our health care system when compared with other nations, but we have called this superiority into question and have been urged to improve health care in America while simultaneously reducing spending—a daunting mission.

One need only to look at other industries to see how technology can improve many of the issues plaguing health care, including both cost and patient outcomes. Improvements in computers and digital imaging along with bandwidth availability and software have made video conferencing in the United States an everyday event. While other industries have rapidly developed and implemented these technologies, health care has been slow to transition to delivery systems that have utilized them. At the University of Arkansas for Medical Sciences (UAMS), we felt in the early 1990s that video-conferencing technologies could provide women's health care across the state of Arkansas and additionally help *improve* women's health care. Over the decades, we have further developed and refined these technologies to address the rural/urban health care disparity, with success. The UAMS Institute for Digital Health and Innovation High Risk Pregnancy Program has led this field nationwide, but we have watched the development of many other groups that have developed related technology-driven programs to improve the lives of women around America.

Obstet Gynecol Clin N Am 47 (2020) xv–xvi
https://doi.org/10.1016/j.ogc.2020.03.001
0889-8545/20/© 2020 Published by Elsevier Inc.

In this issue, we have asked health care professionals to report on various activities that improve women's health care through digital technologies. Topics range from an article defining digital health and its general importance in obstetrics and gynecology to articles on specific subjects, such as telemedicine, in both high- and low-risk obstetrics and telemedicine use for specialty areas, such as gynecologic oncology and maternal psychiatry. We expect that these articles will be stimulating, and we feel that they may help set the stage for far greater uses of these emerging technologies—uses that will further help health care costs and patient care quality.

We had a large support system in reviewing the articles in this issue. Special thanks to Terri Imus, Rosalyn Perkins, Everett Magann, Kristen Zorn, William Greenfield, Wendy Ross, Rachel Armes, and Monica Davidson for their careful review of select articles.

Curtis Lowery, MD
University of Arkansas for
Medical Sciences
Institute for Digital Health and
& Innovation
4301 West Markham Street
Slot 518
Little Rock, AR 72205, USA

E-mail address:
Lowerycurtisl@uams.edu

What Is Digital Health and What Do I Need to Know About It?

Curtis Lowery, MD

KEYWORDS

- Digital health • Telehealth • Telemedicine • mHealth • Remote patient monitoring
- Data analytics • Social media • Obstetrics and gynecology

KEY POINTS

- Digital health technologies improve outcomes within many health care fields, including obstetrics and gynecology.
- Digital health includes telemedicine and telehealth, remote patient monitoring, mobile health applications, data analytics, and social networking.
- Patients, providers, and insurers alike benefit from digital health, with time and cost savings as well as benefits, such as access to aggregate data, which can be utilized to predict disease and outcomes, allowing tailored solutions.
- Some of the essentials of digital health implementation include champion providers, patients in need, technology, peer support system, understanding of laws and regulations, seed funding, and sustainability.
- Ultimately, digital health can help pave the way to a more value-based, direct-to-consumer form of health care.

INTRODUCTION

Digital health represents new technology-driven and data-driven approaches to monitoring and improving patient and population health. Digital health transforms how medicine is delivered and managed: instead of relying on the acute, episodic collection of health information at doctor visits, digital health technologies offer a more comprehensive portrait of an individual patient's health by offering new access to care and greatly enhanced monitoring outside the clinic visit. When these data are aggregated, analyzed, and interpreted, digital health can lead to health strategies that can be applied to entire populations. The digital health scope includes

Telemedicine and telehealth
Remote patient monitoring

Department of Obstetrics and Gynecology, University of Arkansas for Medical Sciences, Institute of Digital Health and Innovation, 4301 West Markham Street Slot 518, Little Rock, AR 72205, USA
E-mail address: LOWERYCURTISL@UAMS.EDU

Obstet Gynecol Clin N Am 47 (2020) 215–225
https://doi.org/10.1016/j.ogc.2020.02.011
0889-8545/20/© 2020 Elsevier Inc. All rights reserved.

obgyn.theclinics.com

Health care mobile applications
Individual-level and population-level data analysis
Social networking

As the US Food and Drug Administration explains, digital health seeks to reduce inefficiencies, improve access, reduce costs, increase quality, and further personalize medicine.[1] The benefits come from empowering patients to seek needed care and track ongoing wellness through technology and for providers to use this information in meaningful ways to deliver precision care to their patients. Society, in turn, benefits from new understandings in preventive care and population health.

DISCUSSION

Digital health technologies enrich the obstetrics and gynecology field, helping improve outcomes for mothers and infants through several delivery modes.

Store-and-Forward

Store-and-forward telehealth technology allows for the transmission of prerecorded health data from one health provider to another, typically to aid with diagnoses or specialty care.[2] Images from tests, such as echocardiograms, computed topography, ultrasounds, and radiographs, often are transferred, as are other digital images and prerecorded videos. Store-and-forward technologies help increase health care efficiency through removing the need to coordinate provider schedules, a common issue when arranging sometimes necessary live video consultations.

Live, Interactive Video

Live, interactive video allows for real-time telemedicine consultations through video and display devices. Video devices include videoconferencing units and Web cameras, whereas display devices include computer monitors, television screens, and even tablet and cell phone screens. In obstetrics and gynecology, real-time video consultations allow patients to see medical providers without leaving their hometown, primary hospital, or even home. This is especially beneficial to rural, medically underserved patients who otherwise might not seek care due to financial and travel constraints.

Live, interactive telemedicine often is used to care for high-risk, rural pregnant women. These high-risk women often have current or past conditions, such as diabetes, obesity, high blood pressure, and blood clots.[3] As part of this high-risk obstetric care, maternal-fetal medicine specialists often consult with distant patients and their providers, offering specialty care that often is restricted to urban and resource-rich areas. During one of these consults, a specialist at a hub (distant) site is able to interact with the patient and her provider at a spoke (originating) site. In addition to basic interaction, such as talking, the specialist is able to view live ultrasounds and other information, such as blood pressure, fundal height, and fetal heart rate. In an emergency, use of video devices can connect experts to rural patients, allowing for quick, lifesaving decisions. With increased access to specialty care comes a decrease in health disparities for high-risk, rural pregnant women and their infants for measures, such as maternal and infant mortality.

High-risk telemedicine consults, such as these, often occur within health facilities. At-home digital health care is becoming more common,[4] however, and some patients, especially those who are lower risk, utilize live video consultation from the comfort of their own homes. This is seen in prenatal care, postdischarge follow-up care, and even lactation support. Even low-risk women are seen frequently for their pregnancies, and interactive telemedicine gives them a more cost-effective and efficient way of receiving care, leading to greater patient satisfaction. Within this model of care, women are taught to collect measures, such as weight, fundal height, blood pressure, and fetal heart rate.[5] Between in-person appointments, medical professionals collect these measures from patients during live video consults and through additional forms of telemedical communication, such as text.

Postdischarge, women must return to health care facilities for postpartum follow-up care. Live video consults help make this process more efficient, allowing new mothers easily accessible care at their fingertips, whereas otherwise they would have to plan to visit their doctor, often with newborns and possibly from a great distance. This saves time, saves money, and reduces stress, which are important for new mothers, who already are stretched thin much of the time.

Lactation support through interactive video is becoming more common. A convenient option for busy, recovering mothers, telelactation offers access to live video consults for immediate or near-immediate problem solving that may help avoid early weaning or unnecessary formula supplementation.[6] This option is even more appealing because virtual, outpatient visits tend to be less expensive than in-person services.

Within gynecology, telecolposcopy offers distant colposcopic examinations through live video for women who have received abnormal Pap smears. In one model, a distant, expert colposcopist guides the onsite colposcopist through the examination, helping to determine if biopsy is needed.[7] Like many telehealth initiatives, telecolposcopy programs help reduce disparities through increased access to health care that may be otherwise unavailable or difficult to obtain for rural, underserved areas.

Mobile Health

With approximately 80% of all American women owning smartphones,[8] mobile health (mHealth) is a promising way to deliver women's health care, and previous studies support this.[9] In family planning and preconception care, mobile applications have shown promising effects on pregnancy outcomes in women with diabetes mellitus, helping to solve problems, such as busy clinics and lack of resources.[10] Furthermore, educational mHealth apps also exist for clinicians and students so that they know what to cover for preconception and family planning care.[11] Another technological preconception tool that can be delivered via mobile device focuses on African American disparities in reproductive health care, helping to close the gap in racial differences.[12]

mHealth apps additionally benefit pregnant women, helping promote management and improvement of areas, such as physical, oral, and mental health wellness. Although some of these apps have not undergone complete trial testing, they show promise. For example, an app for promoting healthy weight gain, diet, and physical activity during pregnancy currently is undergoing testing.[13] Although little is known in the literature about the efficacy of this type of app for physical activity, the literature does show that mHealth has improved service delivery and patient engagement among pregnant women with symptoms of depression.[14] Additionally, another study shows that an oral health promotion app may assist providers when implementing prenatal oral health guidelines, where significant gaps currently exist.[15] This app potentially can improve maternal and infant outcomes, because poor maternal oral health in pregnancy is linked to adverse outcomes for both them and their children.

Social Media

Day-to-day life has become so entwined with social media use that it should be little to no surprise that providers and patients alike find it useful for health care reasons. A survey found that 65% of 4000 polled physicians use social media professionally, including for patient and community interaction.[17] Additionally there are social media sites for medical professionals that are protected from lay audiences, allowing for professionals to safely discuss patient treatment and to ask peers for advice. Other social networking opportunities for physicians include blogs; microblogs, such as Twitter; and media sharing sites, such as YouTube. Although there is still resistance among physicians to utilize social media to interact with patients, some studies show that physicians are developing an interest in online patient interaction with the belief that it may lead to "better education, increased compliance, and better outcomes"[16] for patients.

Risky limitations still exist, however, for physicians' professional use of social media, including poor quality and unreliability of information.[17] For example, supplied medical information may be unreferenced or altogether incomplete, sometimes by poorly identified individuals who lack credibility. There additionally are concerns regarding Health Insurance Portability and Accountability Act compliance, patient-provider boundary violations, licensing issues, and legal issues. Physicians, therefore, should research their options carefully when considering professional social media usage, given the sensitivity surrounding the subject.

Patients, however, have fewer limitations when exploring the health benefits of social media use. Within women's health, patients find positive connections online that help give them essential support that otherwise may be unavailable to them.[18] This virtual connection often is seen among childbearing women who use social networking for emotional support and additionally to help them make parenting decisions. One exploratory study shows that new mothers who blog feel a sense of connection to family and friends that they otherwise may not have, having a positive impact on maternal well-being, as measured by parenting stress, couple conflict, marital satisfaction, and depression.[19] These improvements in maternal well-being through social support also are linked to improved child outcomes.

Remote Patient Monitoring

Remote monitoring is becoming more common as digital health technologies continue to develop. This type of real-time monitoring occurs when technology, often wearable devices or cell phones, is used to collect health data from patients and then transmit that data to health care providers at another location. Patients who are monitored remotely sometimes are at home and other times at another care facility—or, they might even wear the monitoring device wherever they need to go, be that home, work, the grocery store, the gym, and so forth. This may be the case for instances, such as looking for abnormal heart rate. Remote monitoring within ambulances reduces time to treatment and allows for emergency teams to be better prepared on patient arrival.[20] Overall, it shows promise for present and future health care delivery through reducing costs, travel time, and need for physical appointments at health care facilities, freeing space for those who need it most.

Data Analytics

Big data has become today's gold rush, offering many fields—including retail, child welfare, the justice system, and medicine—an opportunity to collect and analyze large sets of aggregate data. This, in turn, allows professionals to tailor solutions not only to problems that are evident and present[21] but also to problems that are predicted. In the health care field, this ability to predict outcomes and possible future disease allows for increased, targeted prevention.[22] The American College of Obstetricians and Gynecologists (ACOG) leads several projects within their Health Informatics Department that support data-driven solutions in women's health, including[23]

- ACOG Prenatal Record integrates the ACOG clinical guidelines with electronic health record systems to provide clinical documentation and improved obstetrics/gynecologic workflow.
- The Birth Registry by ACOG is a clinical data registry that captures labor and delivery data, proving information about maternal health outcomes that can aid quality improvement.
- The Family Planning Annual Report Interoperability Initiative is a reporting system that collects reproductive health data from Title X sites across the nation.
- Women's Health Registry Alliance is a central data warehouse, preventing data silos, which aims to improve women's health outcomes.

Digital Health Benefits

There are many rich benefits to integrating digital health into society. One of the most overarching benefits is that, simply, patient outcomes are improved through more efficient, easily accessible health care. Digital health has a positive impact on patients, providers, and insurers alike.

Patients[24]
- Reduces and sometimes eliminates travel time
- Reduces costs through less travel
- Improves time away from work and other responsibilities, such as child care
- Reduces exposure to other potentially contagious patients
- Improves continuity of care through utilizing data registries/warehouses and electronic health records
- Reduces unnecessary patient transports
- Reduces unnecessary emergency department and urgent care visits by offering around-the-clock access on smart devices
- Improves outcomes through data analytics and targeted solutions/prevention

Providers/Hospitals[25]
- Supports risk-based financial models through telehealth-supplemented care
- Reduces hospital readmissions
- Improves patient follow-through and fewer missed appointments
- Prevents health issues
- Increases revenue—video visits decrease the time of each encounter, allowing providers to see more patients
- Allows providers to treat and monitor remote patients 24/7
- Allows for private payer reimbursement
- Provides access to aggregate data

Insurers[25]
- Helps insurers reach more patients
- Allows insurers to extend health care to rural, underserved areas
- Allows insurers to supplement health care
- Potentially helps insurers meet network adequacy standards
- Provides access to aggregate data

Planning, launching, and sustaining a digital health program can be daunting, but there are good resources available for guidance. Some of the digital health essentials include

- Champion providers
- Patients in need
- Technology (secure network, equipment and/or software, and staff to troubleshoot)
- Peer support system (successful programs and telehealth resource centers [TRCs])
- Understanding of laws and regulations
- Seed funding (grants)
- Sustainability (reimbursement, contracts)

Champion Providers

It can be challenging to find providers who are willing to integrate digital health into their practices. It is imperative, however, to find providers who not only will embrace digital health but also who will be champions for it. These champions will be those who lead digital health initiatives and who push for updated laws and regulations that support digital health.

Patients in Need

Just like any health care program, digital health programs require patients who need the services. Digital health particularly benefits rural and medically underserved patients or those who have difficulty leaving their homes for care. Digital health benefits many urban residents, however, as well, although this is mainly a convenience factor. For instance, someone who resides in the city and who does not lack access to care may enjoy the convenience of attending an appointment without having to leave the workplace.

For rural and medically underserved patients, digital health sometimes makes the difference between receiving care and going without it. It has been known to reduce critical barriers to health care, reducing health disparities and improving patient outcomes.

Technology

Digital health requires digital technology. For telehealth and remote patient monitoring, providers must utilize a secure telehealth network, equipment and/or software, and staff to troubleshoot. Technology components include clinical carts, nonclinical carts, desktop units, room systems, and peripherals, such as blood pressure monitors and scopes (**Fig. 1**).

Peer Support Systems

TRCs assist organizations and individuals who provide or are interested in providing digital health, in particular telehealth.[26] Generally, this assistance is free of charge thanks to federal funding and includes education and technical assistance, along with other resources (**Fig. 2**). Each regional TRC caters specifically to its region's needs. The National Consortium of Telehealth Resource Centers works to provide[26]

- A central Web site
- Monthly national webinars
- Presentations and representation at conferences
- Position statements and templates

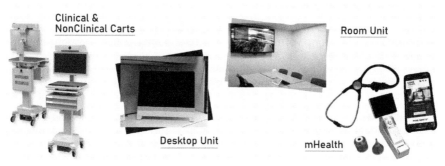

Fig. 1. Telehealth technology components.

- Collaborative grant proposals and projects
- A collective brain trust of resources and information

Understanding Laws and Regulations

One of the most overwhelming, yet essential, aspects of practicing digital health is understanding the various associated laws and regulations. Credentialing and licensure requirements and processes are cumbersome particularly for telehealth providers, especially considering telehealth providers must be licensed and credentialed at a patient's location, which is sometimes out of state. It is imperative also to become familiarized with state telehealth parity laws, because the existence of one for a state means that telehealth services are equally reimbursed in comparison to the same services offered in person.

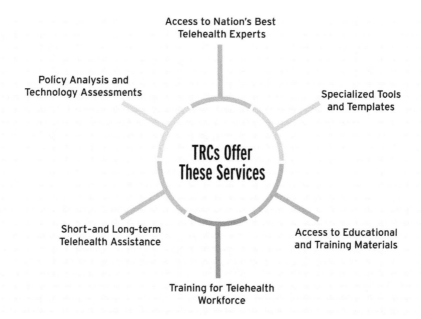

Fig. 2. Services offered by TRCs. (*Data from* The National Consortium of Telehealth Resource Centers. Available at: https://www.telehealthresourcecenter.org/.)

Seed Funding and Sustainability

Seed funding is important when beginning a digital health program, and there are many grants and other forms of assistance available for this purpose through both federal and nonfederal resources. Federal funding often is available for telehealth and related technological solutions through entities, such as the Health Resources and Services Administration, the US Department of Agriculture, the National Institutes for Health, and the Substance Abuse and Mental Health Services Administration. Additionally, reliable broadband is essential to any digital health initiative. The Universal Service Administrative Co. (USAC) helps support rural broadband needs through their Rural Health Care Program.[27] Through the USAC Healthcare Connect Fund Program, awarded health care providers and consortia receive a flat 65% discount on broadband expenses and network equipment.

Financially sustaining digital health programs can be tricky, but it is entirely possible. Membership fees help sustain programs, and sometimes grant funding is necessary to sustain a program. Parity laws, such as the ones for telehealth services, also are important for sustainability. Collaborative measures, including contracts between physician groups and insurance companies, are necessary for sustainability in states where parity does not exist.

Future of Digital Health

The future of digital health within obstetrics and gynecology includes expanding into home-based and direct-to-consumer care. This will include live video consults, remote patient monitoring, and mHealth. Although these methods already are used within obstetrics and gynecology, the future will bring common usage of digital health technologies outside of the clinical environment. Mobile apps especially show some promise, due to their popularity: as of early 2018, there were more than 300,000 health apps available worldwide, nearly double that of 2015.[28] More than 200 apps are added each day. The uptick in mHealth use has led to promising obstetrics and gynecology apps, such as those for mobile ultrasound that allow health care providers to view scans in real-time at the point of care, wherever that may be.[29]

Health care is shifting to a value-based model from the current standard, which is fee for service. Value-based care is exactly what its name implies—health care that focuses on quality of health care services versus quantity. Under value-based health care, providers are paid based on patient health outcomes instead of being paid on the amount of health care services that they deliver.[30] Digital health often is an investment upfront, but it supports value-based care by streamlining health care and creating lower costs and better outcomes down the line.[31]

SUMMARY

Digital health technologies improve outcomes within many health care fields, including obstetrics and gynecology. They include telemedicine and telehealth, remote patient monitoring, mHealth applications, data analytics, and social networking. Patients, providers, and insurers alike benefit from digital health, with time and cost savings as well as benefits, such as access to aggregate data, which can be utilized to predict disease and outcomes, allowing tailored solutions.

Some of the essentials of digital health implementation include champion providers, patients in need, technology (secure network, equipment, and/or software and staff to troubleshoot), peer support systems (successful programs and TRCs), understanding of laws and regulations, seed funding (grants), and sustainability (reimbursement and contracts). Within this framework, successful programs can and will be established, leading health care into a more value-based future that is largely focused on direct-to-consumer care.

DISCLOSURE

The author has nothing to disclose.

REFERENCES

1. USDA. USDA. Available at: https://www.usda.gov/. Accessed September 30, 2019.
2. About Telehealth. Available at: https://www.cchpca.org/about/about-telehealth/store-and-forward-asynchronous. Accessed September 30, 2019.
3. High-Risk Pregnancy. Eunice Kennedy Shriver National Institute of Child Health and Human Development. Available at: https://www.nichd.nih.gov/health/topics/high-risk. Accessed September 30, 2019.
4. Wade VA, Karnon J, Elshaug AG, et al. A systematic review of economic analyses of telehealth services using real time video communication. BMC Health Serv Res 2010;10:233. Available at: https://bmchealthservres.biomedcentral.com/articles/10.1186/1472-6963-10-233. Accessed September 30, 2019.
5. Mooij MJMD, Hodny RL, Oneil DA, et al. OB Nest: Reimagining Low-Risk Prenatal Care. Mayo Clin Proc 2018;93(4):458–66.
6. Uscher-Pines L, Mehrotra A, Bogen DL. The emergence and promise of telelactation. Am J Obstet Gynecol 2017;217(2). https://doi.org/10.1016/j.ajog.2017.04.043.
7. Treating Arkansas Women via Telemedicine. Healthcare Innovation. Available at: https://www.hcinnovationgroup.com/home/article/13019458/treating-arkansas-women-via-telemedicine. Accessed September 30, 2019.
8. Demographics of Mobile Device Ownership and Adoption in the United States. Pew Research Center: Internet, Science & Tech. 2019. Available at: https://www.pewinternet.org/fact-sheet/mobile/. Accessed September 30, 2019.
9. Mehralizade A, Schor S, Coleman CM, et al. Mobile health apps in OB-GYN-embedded psychiatric care: commentary. JMIR Mhealth Uhealth 2017;5(10):e152. Available at: https://www.ncbi.nlm.nih.gov/pmc/articles/PMC5650672/. Accessed September 30, 2019.
10. Nwolise CH, Carey N, Shawe J. Preconception care education for women with diabetes: a systematic review of conventional and digital health interventions. J Med Internet Res 2016;18(11):e291. Available at: https://www.ncbi.nlm.nih.gov/pubmed/27826131. Accessed September 30, 2019.
11. NEW Mobile App: Preconception Care Quick Reference. Before, Between & Beyond Pregnancy. 2018. Available at: https://beforeandbeyond.org/2018/new-mobile-app-preconception-care-quick-reference/. Accessed September 30, 2019.
12. Lyons J. Software seeks to reduce disparities in preconception care: HealthCity. Boston (MA): Boston Medical Center; 2019. Available at: https://www.bmc.org/healthcity/population-health/software-seeks-reduce-disparities-preconception-care. Accessed September 30, 2019.
13. Henriksson P, Sandborg J, Blomberg M, et al. A smartphone app to promote healthy weight gain, diet, and physical activity during pregnancy (HealthyMoms): protocol for a randomized controlled trial. JMIR Res Protoc 2019;8(3):e13011.

Available at: https://www.ncbi.nlm.nih.gov/pubmed/30821695. Accessed September 30, 2019.

14. Hantsoo L, Criniti S, Khan A, et al. A Mobile Application for Monitoring and Management of Depressed Mood in a Vulnerable Pregnant Population. Psychiatr Serv 2018;69(1):104–7. Available at: https://www.ncbi.nlm.nih.gov/pubmed/29032705. Accessed September 30, 2019.

15. Vamos CA, Griner SB, Kirchharr C, et al. The development of a theory-based eHealth app prototype to promote oral health during prenatal care visits. Transl Behav Med 2019;9(6):1100–11. Available at: https://www.ncbi.nlm.nih.gov/pubmed/31009536. Accessed September 30, 2019.

16. Available at: https://books.google.com/books?hl=en&lr=&id=uuZN nyYWK2EC&oi=fnd&pg=PA244&ots=55KFIE1SbD&sig=1N4bcx–Qir2_gmH sDeqe4TYOSs#v=snippet&q=better%20education%2C%20increased%20com pliance%2C%20and%20better%20outcomes&f=false.

17. Ventola CL. Social media and health care professionals: benefits, risks, and best practices. P T 2014;39(7):491–520. Available at: https://www.ncbi.nlm.nih.gov/pmc/articles/PMC4103576/. Accessed September 30, 2019.

18. Gleeson DM, Craswell A, Jones CM. Women's use of social networking sites related to childbearing: An integrative review. Women Birth 2019;32(4): 294–302. Available at: https://www.ncbi.nlm.nih.gov/pubmed/30606628. Accessed September 30, 2019.

19. McDaniel BT, Coyne SM, Holmes EK. New mothers and media use: associations between blogging, social networking, and maternal well-being. Matern Child Health J 2012;16(7):1509–17. SpringerLink. Available at: https://link.springer.com/article/10.1007/s10995-011-0918-2. Accessed September 30, 2019.

20. Meystre S. The current state of telemonitoring: a comment on the literature. Telemed J E Health 2005;11(1):63–9.

21. Erekson EA, Iglesia CB. Improving patient outcomes in gynecology: the role of large data registries and big data analytics. J Minim Invasive Gynecol 2015; 22(7):1124–9. Available at: https://www.ncbi.nlm.nih.gov/pubmed/26188310. Accessed September 30, 2019.

22. Amarasingham R, Patzer RE, Huesch M, et al. Implementing electronic health care predictive analytics: considerations and challenges. Health Aff 2014;33(7): 1148–54. Available at: https://www.healthaffairs.org/doi/full/10.1377/hlthaff.2014.0352. Accessed September 30, 2019.

23. Women's Health Care Physicians. ACOG. Available at: https://www.acog.org/About-ACOG/ACOG-Departments/Health-Information-Technology?IsMobileSet=false. Accessed September 30, 2019.

24. Telemedicine. Telemedicine | Department of Obstetrics & Gynecology. Available at: https://obgyn.wustl.edu/patients/high-risk-pregnancy/telemedicine/. Accessed September 30, 2019.

25. mHealthIntelligence. Can Telehealth Fill Health Insurer's Provider Network Gaps? mHealthIntelligence. 2016. Available at: https://mhealthintelligence.com/news/can-telehealth-fill-health-insurers-provider-network-gaps. Accessed September 30, 2019.

26. National Consortium of Telehealth Research Centers. National Consortium of Telehealth Research Centers. Available at: https://www.telehealthresourcecenter.org/. Accessed September 30, 2019.

27. Rural Health Care. Healthcare connect fund - rural health care program - USAC.org. Available at: https://www.usac.org/rhc/. Accessed September 30, 2019.

28. The Rise of mHealth apps: a market snapshot. Liquid State. 2019. Available at: https://liquid-state.com/mhealth-apps-market-snapshot/. Accessed September 30, 2019.
29. SonoSite. 9 top apps for bedside ultrasound. Emergency Physicians Monthly. Available at: https://epmonthly.com/article/9-top-apps-for-bedside-ultrasound/. Accessed September 30, 2019.
30. NEJM Catalyst. What is value-based healthcare? NEJM Catalyst. 2019. Available at: https://catalyst.nejm.org/what-is-value-based-healthcare/. Accessed September 30, 2019.
31. Cohen JK. Innovation is a value-based care investment, health system CEOs say. Modern Healthcare. 2019. Available at: https://www.modernhealthcare.com/technology/innovation-value-based-care-investment-health-system-ceos-say. Accessed September 30, 2019.

Reframing Telehealth
Regulation, Licensing, and Reimbursement in Connected Care

Janet L. McCauley, MD, MHA, CPC, FACOG[a,b],
Anthony E. Swartz, BS, RT(R), RDMS[b,*]

KEYWORDS

- Telehealth • Telemedicine • Reimbursement • Virtual care • Fee for service
- Value-based care • Connected care • Artificial intelligence

KEY POINTS

- Variation in regulation and professional licensing for telehealth services is driven by existing federal and state-based parameters developed around face-to-face care.
- New hybrid delivery models blending telehealth modalities with face-to-face care remain unaddressed by current regulatory standards, but may be beneficial to accelerate integration of telehealth into traditional workflows.
- Value-based payment methodologies have potential to achieve savings in the total cost of care by rewarding efficiency of remote care delivery and improved outcomes across a population.
- Innovative technology solutions for connected care, such as algorithmic decision support, natural language processing, artificial intelligence, and machine-based learning, will require new regulatory paradigms.
- Additional research concerning the most appropriate clinical and cost-effective use cases is needed to inform regulatory and payment policy, particularly in obstetrics and gynecology.

INTRODUCTION AND BACKGROUND

The advent and adoption of telehealth technologies brings opportunity for increased access, efficiency, and cost-effectiveness of care delivery. Despite its existence for many years with evolution through multiple generations of technology development, use remains highly variable across geographic, state, and health system boundaries within the United States. Although access to technology represents an obvious entry

[a] Blue Cross Blue Shield of North Carolina, PO Box 2291 Durham, NC 27702-2291, USA;
[b] Department of Obstetrics & Gynecology, Duke University School of Medicine, Box 3967, Durham, NC 27710, USA
* Corresponding author.
E-mail address: anthony.swartz@duke.edu

Obstet Gynecol Clin N Am 47 (2020) 227–239
https://doi.org/10.1016/j.ogc.2020.02.001
0889-8545/20/© 2020 Elsevier Inc. All rights reserved.

obgyn.theclinics.com

requirement, regulatory, legal, and reimbursement conditions both facilitate and hinder adoption.[1] These conditions vary across state boundaries, practice settings, patient types, provider types, choice of technology, clinical use cases, and payer source: literally all aspects of care delivery. As a result, patients may or may not have access to virtual care depending on where they are physically located, what service they receive, the type of technology deployed, or who provides their health insurance.

Given a shared goal of communicating accurate information to achieve a desired health outcome, people may wonder how the regulatory and payment environment evolved into its current state of complexity and inconsistency, and how this fragmented environment has affected adoption of virtual care. This article explores the legal, technical, cultural, financial, and care delivery influencers that determine how telehealth is regulated and paid (**Box 1**), with a special focus on how these components shape adoption of telehealth within women's health. By identifying actionable steps that have potential to advance the role of telehealth in appropriate use cases, this article provides context for near and long-term goals to better realize the added value of connected care to traditional care delivery.

THE DRIVERS OF REGULATION AND PAYMENT
What Is Telehealth?

The definition of telehealth has varied over time and across organizations. In their 1996 guide to telehealth, the Institute of Medicine (IOM) defined telehealth as:

> the use of electronic information and communications technologies to provide and support health care when distance separates participants.[2]

The following year, the World Health Organization (WHO) adopted this more expanded definition:

> The delivery of health care services, where distance is a critical factor, by all health care professionals using information and communication technologies for the exchange of valid information for diagnosis, treatment and prevention of disease and

---

Box 1
The drivers of regulation and payment

- Definitions of telehealth
- Technical delivery
  - Modality
  - Data accuracy
  - Data exchange
  - Privacy and security
- Clinical encounter
  - Provider of service
  - Recipient of service
  - Setting and location
- Reimbursement
- Evidence for clinical use and cost

Opportunities in women's telehealth services

Pathways forward: the twenty-first century telehealth ecosystem

Beyond the limitations: summary and steps forward.

injuries, research and evaluation, and for the continuing education of health care providers, all in the interests of advancing the health of individuals and their communities.[3]

Most state laws governing the practice of telehealth include a definition for telehealth or telemedicine in the statute. These definitions are varied, but one similarity they all share is that they are open to interpretation, which can create inconsistency in subsequent rules, regulations, and payment policy. As an example, distance requirements found in state laws are variably stated as "sufficient distance," or specific mileage requirements, or nonspecifically as "distance."[4] With rapid innovation in technology, definitions incorporated into statute may become rapidly outdated, and require additional legislation to change.

Technical Delivery

Most implementations of telehealth are in one of several categories, including data store/data store and forward, direct patient interaction, remote patient monitoring, and hybrid or combination (**Table 1**).

Data store or store and forward refers to patient-entered data parameters that are stored and later accessed, or forwarded to a clinician for subsequent analysis. Remote monitoring may involve transmission of physiologic data, such as continuous glucose monitoring, cardiac rhythm tracking, or blood pressure monitoring.

An area of interest in women's health that is not represented in the literature or by current regulation is a hybrid telehealth model that integrates traditional care delivery systems, teleradiology, and telehealth systems. Teleradiology is one of the first use cases to be adopted as a telehealth platform. However, traditionally teleradiology did not include synchronous patient interactions or real-time video feed from the modality. Women's health and prenatal diagnosis are well suited to a model that combines real-time video interaction between image interpreting providers, clinical care providers, and patients. This hybrid model leverages both traditional teleradiology platforms and newer telehealth systems that permit remote patient and clinician interactions via video as well as real-time video feed from the ultrasonography modality. Given that regulation and reimbursement policies are often specific to modality, it remains to be determined how hybrid models that blend multiple modalities would be treated.

Data accuracy and technical quality play important roles in the success of telehealth. At present, technical performance of telemonitoring devices is subject to the same US Food and Drug Administration (FDA) approval pathways as direct patient care devices. Despite intent to protect users from harm, devices have been marketed

Table 1	
Telehealth categories and use case implementations	
Telehealth Category	**Typical Implementations**
Data store/forward	Asynchronous patient encounter, synchronous telehealth encounter/consult, or subsequent future encounters
Direct patient interaction	Real-time patient encounters or asynchronous encounters
Remote monitoring	Real-time, store and forward, wearable and mobile operating systems, prenatal care
Hybrid/combination	Prenatal diagnosis, remote antenatal monitoring

and sold without clear indicators of data accuracy or that data transferred is sufficient for sound clinical judgment.[5] Nevertheless, remote monitoring and reporting devices are increasingly prevalent. In anticipation of an evolving need to evaluate device performance and effectiveness, the FDA has created the National Evaluation System for Health Technology to accelerate the timely assimilation of information needed for regulatory decision making.[6] Novel processes to collate information around device-generated data and subsequent clinical outcomes will provide accountability for the technical limitations of these devices, their proliferation, and the reliability of data they collect and transmit.

Data exchange is another area that warrants innovative regulation. The Meaningful Use regulations require that health care providers and organizations link patients to their health information, but there is no guidance or standard pathway for patients to self-direct transfer of health information[7] from their personal devices to distinctly separate telemedicine systems that may differ from the originating source of the health information. Application programming interfaces (APIs) are commonly used to transfer data between 2 different Web applications. Similar applications of APIs will be required to facilitate patient-directed transfer of protected health information data. With increasing mobility among Americans and their readiness to cross geographic boundaries, this use case is likely the next frontier for innovation in telehealth.

Mandl and Kohane note[7] that, although the Health Insurance Portability and Accountability Act of 1996 (HIPAA) mandates provision of health data to patients, health care organizations frequently cite HIPAA concerns as a reason to restrict health information availability. These concerns may reflect the fear associated with data security once health information is no longer exclusively under the control of the originating organization. The role of HIPAA compliance, including data security, is mostly handled by technology solution providers. However, the organization delivering the telehealth service must properly validate adequate security of its own internal networks, as well as adequately validate solution or technology vendor compliance with applicable state and federal security guidelines.

The Clinical Encounter

The most straightforward application of telehealth serves as a direct substitute for the face-to-face patient encounter. In their 2016 survey of physicians performing direct patient care, the American Medical Association (AMA) notes that live interactive video-conferencing was used by 12.6% of physicians and was the modality with most prevalent use.[8] Of all telehealth modalities, videoconferencing is most similar to traditional face-to-face encounters for diagnosis and treatment, and is the most common modality subject to regulation and payment policy. In 2018, the Center for Connected Health Policy (CCHP) noted all states except 1 providing Medicaid reimbursement for live audiovisual encounters, compared with 20 states providing reimbursement for remote patient monitoring, and very few defining and reimbursing asynchronous store-and-forward technology.[4]

The live interactive modality also assumes that professional providers conduct clinical services similar to in-person encounters for assimilation of information, medical decision making, and documentation. Fundamentally, telehealth is still the practice of medicine, nursing, and other clinical professions, only with the assistance of remote technology as a communication tool. Governance of the practice of telehealth as a professional service remains under the purview of various licensing boards whose rules and foundation are again based on traditional face-to-face care. At present, these rules continue to reside in the respective states where the practitioner holds a license, in the form of state statute and regulatory board policy and enforcement. Factors regarding clinical practice that may be included in state-based oversight include:

- Location of the patient
- Standard of care
- Provider-patient relationship
- Prescribing
- Documentation in permanent record
- Appropriate training
- Ethical standards
- Medicolegal risk

Most states consider the practice of medicine, and thus the practice of telehealth, to occur in the state where the patient is located, regardless of the location of the provider or state of residence of the patient. However, location of the provider is also addressed in some state laws. Alaska passed legislation in 2016 (SB0098C) that enabled an Alaska-licensed provider in another state to prescribe for patients within Alaska without first conducting a physical examination, thus removing the requirement for the provider to also be located in the state.[9] This decision was supported by an unexpected regulator, the Federal Trade Commission (FTC), who viewed the ruling as procompetitive and likely to enhance access to care with reduced costs in a state with underserved populations, limited numbers of providers, and geographic constraints.[10]

Given the ease with which patients cross state boundaries as part of their daily personal and professional lives, mapping of practitioner licensure to location of the patient remains a logistical challenge in telehealth, and in particular for providers who normally render face-to-face care to their patients. The Interstate Medical Licensure Compact seeks to alleviate this challenge by providing an agreement among 29 states, District of Columbia, and Guam, whereby physicians may acquire licensure and practice across state lines within the compact if they meet eligibility requirements based on primary state of residence, training, and background check.[11] In 2019, Florida passed progressive legislation that allows health professionals licensed out of state, but without a Florida license, to deliver telehealth services to Florida patients when specific criteria are met, such as registration with the Florida Department of Health and prohibition against providing in-person services within the state.[12]

Establishing a provider-patient relationship is another function traditionally mandated by statute or overseen by state licensing boards. Debate continues as to whether and how a professional relationship may be established through a virtual encounter. In 2018, the AMA surveyed all 50 states, finding that all states allow physicians to establish relationships with new patients by telehealth, but that restrictions exist in various caveats, such as setting or modality.[13]

Exceptions to broader positions on establishing a provider-patient relationship via virtual care exist, most notably in prescribing, with particular caution in prescribing of controlled substances. In their 2019 revised policy for access to behavioral telehealth services, Massachusetts Medicaid (MassHealth) requires an initial in-person examination before prescribing schedule II controlled substances by telehealth, with an additional requirement for ongoing in-person examinations every 3 months for the duration of prescription of the schedule II controlled substance.[14] Although the policy opens certain behavioral health and substance abuse services to MassHealth members via telehealth, the recurring in-person examination requirement represents a higher standard than the federal Ryan Haight Act of 2008, which was originally intended to prevent Internet pharmacies from selling controlled substances online.[15]

In addition, the revised MassHealth policy includes requirements for documentation of best practices and training protocols that form a higher standard than state medical board and other payer requirements.

In setting regulatory policy, much debate focuses on whether all services and diagnoses available for face-to-face care are appropriate for telehealth. The AMA's position on Ethical Practice in Telemedicine[16] holds physicians responsible to the same standards of professionalism in diagnosis and treatment during virtual care episodes, thus setting a standard for equivalency. In response, many specialty societies have developed practice guidelines, position statements, and toolkits to guide their memberships.[17,18] State medical boards may also support professional judgment by allowing provider discretion in deciding whether adequate information for diagnosis and treatment may be obtained without in-person evaluation, or if circumstances require initiation of a face-to-face encounter.

In addition, medical malpractice risk in telehealth may arise from regulatory and jurisdictional gaps. In a 2014 national survey of family practitioners, Moore and colleagues[19] noted that 41% of respondents expressed liability concerns as a barrier to telehealth use, secondary to lack of training, reimbursement, and cost of equipment. Uncertain venues for data-assisted diagnosis, unclear understanding of which states govern medical practice in a remote encounter, lack of legal opinions, statutory variation in caps on damages, and inability of liability carriers to assess financial risk all contribute to potential exposure.[20]

How Is Telehealth Reimbursed?

Similar to issues regarding oversight and state regulation of remote clinical practice, telehealth reimbursement struggles to find its place in a system built around face-to-face care. Despite professional society guidance regarding appropriateness of services potentially rendered via telehealth, legislation and downstream payment policy continue to drive telehealth service coverage concerning an array of circumstances, including medical conditions, provider type, patient type, setting, and frequency of encounters. Over time, restrictions over circumstances such as these have tended to ease, but inconsistently across localities and payer sources.

Of all service types, behavioral health represents the most common clinical service for expanded coverage. Behavioral health makes a compelling telehealth use case for at least 2 reasons: limited access in many localities, and apparent similarities to face-to-face care delivery by lack of need for hands-on examination. In their 2017 gap analysis of Medicaid coverage,[21] the American Telemedicine Association notes that all states have coverage and reimbursement for behavioral health services via live video consultation, although specifics of these laws vary. However, how does service parity relate to equivalent payment?

Telehealth is typically reimbursed through the same codes reported for in-person fee-for-service payment. Most of these service codes were created based on vignettes excerpted from typical face-to-face scenarios, describing the work to perform the service in person. Service code valuation is then based on resource consumption and unique work, which the Centers for Medicare and Medicaid Services (CMS) with input from the AMA determines by assigning relative value units to components of physician work, practice expense, and professional liability insurance.[22]

Documentation of required key components for history and physical examination or time requirements represents an additional hurdle in translating face-to-face to virtual service coding. Resource-based valuation and documentation requirements of existing codes thus both create a problematic payment methodology for fee-for-service virtual care by emphasizing the acquisition cost of technology and potentially irrelevant face-to-face workflows.

In response to increasing demand for virtual encounters, CMS and the AMA have created additional service codes specific to telehealth, along with modifiers and place-of-service designations to identify a claim resulting from a remote encounter. In 2018, CMS also proposed changes to the Medicare Physician Fee Schedule in an attempt to reduce the burden of documentation and complexity of payment for outpatient/office Evaluation & Management services, by allowing new and established visits the option to be documented solely by medical decision making or time.[23] Better availability of specific codes, in conjunction with relief of documentation requirements for detailed elements of history and physical examination, could align these codes to better report telehealth encounters. However, additional granularity in fee-for-service telehealth coding apart from existing face-to-face codes may perpetuate telehealth as a separate and parallel system for service capture and payment.

The value in telehealth lies not in the reimbursement associated with a specific telehealth encounter but in tying virtual care to reduced resources for care delivery and downstream clinical results. Alternative payment models (APMs) provide an opportunity for goal alignment around access, improved outcomes, patient experience, care coordination, and reduced total cost of care. Nussbaum and colleagues[24] established a 4-step foundational framework for maturity of APMs:

1. Fee for service, no link to quality and value
2. Fee for service, link to quality and value
3. Fee-for-service APMs, with upside gainsharing ± downside risk
4. Condition-specific or comprehensive population-based payment

Compared with fee for service, APMs reward efficiency rather than volume of care. Value frameworks position telehealth as a communication tool to achieve an outcome across a population, rather than a substitute for face-to-face care coupled with fee for service reimbursement on a per-use basis.

Development of a value-based framework requires testing not only of the financial models but of the care delivery and integrated workflows that are inherent to value-based care. For example, in their 2018 report to Congress, the CMS and Center for Medicare and Medicaid Innovation noted enhanced telehealth benefits for asynchronous dermatology and ophthalmology within the Next Generation Accountable Care Organization Model, beyond those under original Medicare.[25] Participants have the opportunity to accept more financial risk than those under other Accountable Care Organization programs but also have the opportunity to select flexible payment options that support infrastructure and work flow process improvement relevant to telehealth. Results from these model programs will be important to inform both care delivery and payment models for telehealth.

What Is the Evidence for the Most Appropriate Clinical Use Cases and Cost Scenarios?

A final contributor to inconsistent regulation and payment policy in telehealth is the lack of agreement regarding the most effective use cases, their impact on total cost of care, and their scalability. In their systematic review of evidence for telehealth, the Agency for Healthcare Research and Quality (AHRQ) identified higher rates of published evidence for remote monitoring for chronic conditions, and behavioral health communication and counseling.[26] Evidence is inconsistent in both quantity and quality and is highly dependent on research methodology and care setting. Additional evidence is needed in 4 distinct capacities:

1. Validation of accuracy of remote monitoring technology, as discussed earlier
2. Clinical effectiveness of the remote intervention versus traditional care
3. Patient and provider experience, including ease of use
4. Demonstration of equivalent or lower cost of care

Results of randomized controlled trials testing telemonitoring and telemessaging have been mixed, some suggesting additional evaluation before widespread dissemination of telemonitoring technology for chronic disease management.[27] In their commentary on telehealth in heart failure, Fraiche and colleagues[28] advocate for large-scale pragmatic trials to overcome the challenges of extrapolating fragmented evidence from controlled trials set in different health systems and regulatory environments.

Legislated through the Patient Protection and Affordable Care Act (ACA) of 2010, the Patient-Centered Outcomes Research Institute (PCORI) funds numerous pragmatic comparative clinical effectiveness research trials, with focus on patient experience. They have identified telehealth as a member-centric tool with potential to engage patients in proactive health management.[29] Examples of PCORI-funded telehealth research published on their Web site show improved access from enhanced behavioral health referral processes in a pediatric population, and clinical equivalence to in-person care through asynchronous teledermatology for patients with psoriasis.

The impact of telehealth services on total cost of care represents an area of growing research interest, with direct implications for regulatory and payment policy decisions. Telehealth is reported to reduce costs by enabling more efficient resource use at the practice level,[30] but the convenience of direct-to-consumer models may increase use, thereby potentially increasing costs in fee-for-service models.[31] However, Anderson and colleagues[32] reported total cost savings in a fee-for-service population following asynchronous E-consults in lieu of face-to-face cardiology referrals, although they noted that such analyses are infrequently performed and reported.

Although research efforts are increasing in number and in designs that can be extrapolated across larger populations, uncertainty limits the ability to scale results and invest in needed processes and technology across health systems and jurisdictions. Numerous pilot programs and telehealth program innovations are available for benchmarking, most notably the increasing prevalence of telehealth solutions for care management initiated through the US Department of Veterans Affairs,[33] but national or regional care delivery and payment models are not always translatable to local systems. Inability to accurately predict clinical and financial outcomes is also a potential driver of increased regulatory and payment oversight, because of concerns of increased cost risk coupled with nominal or neutral clinical benefit.

OPPORTUNITIES IN WOMEN'S TELEHEALTH SERVICES

Despite promising preliminary data for telehealth adoption in women's health, uptake has been limited. In their report of a 2016 AMA survey across specialties, modalities, and practice types, Kane and Gillis[34] found telehealth use for obstetricians-gynecologists lower than the average across all specialties and for all modalities, and lower than that reported for all other surgical specialties. Because of existing research focus around behavioral health and chronic disease management, it is expected that literature supporting use cases within women's health delivery is less prevalent, thus potentially explaining lower adoption rates. Lack of available remote monitoring technology with minimal patient interaction may also contribute to underuse.

Developing evidence for effective use cases specific to women's health is thus necessary to provide frameworks that will guide emerging regulatory and payment models. Several recent evaluations add to this body of evidence. These evaluative models share an integrated approach, using technology as a communication tool embedded in face-to-face workflows, patient centricity, and support of evidence-based care. A recent systematic review of evidence for telehealth interventions for low-risk and high-risk obstetrics and family planning populations found positive effect related to several interventions, such as text messaging to support breastfeeding and smoking cessation.[35]

In addition to patients as recipients of care, other recipients within women's health care include family members of patients, groups of patients and family caregivers, as well as other medical professionals and medical consultants. Recent developments in telehealth technologies enable multiple medical providers and consultants to interact with a single patient or groups of patients simultaneously. This multipresence concept may be leveraged for mass patient education activities in real time. Additional capabilities such as screen-sharing, or content push technologies enable care providers to share and annotate content with patients in real time for consultation, care coordination, and patient education. Although feasible for emerging care and education models, pathways to achieve multipresence telehealth concepts require reevaluation of existing regulation around patient-provider relationships and health plan benefits limiting coverage to groups of beneficiaries.

PATHWAYS FORWARD: THE TWENTY-FIRST CENTURY TELEHEALTH ECOSYSTEM

In modern medicine, the potential for connected care reaches beyond extension of in-person encounters with a traditional provider who is licensed and credentialed to perform face-to-face care. Telehealth as a mechanism for indirect patient care represents a paradigm shift in care delivery. Data gathering from remote monitoring and storage at the individual level may be used to benefit individuals, or may be combined into a larger dataset or registry to encompass a population of patients. These data could then be analyzed for research purposes or population health management, ultimately returning to utility for another individual patient's care. Artificial intelligence and algorithmic analyses using consolidated data may also guide real-time medical decision making for individual patients.

The growth of medical devices and decision support tools based on aggregated patient data is innovative but has created a new need for regulatory oversight, in which the distinction of who delivers care, who makes medical decisions, and the role of third parties becomes blurred. Medical algorithms within devices are often nontransparent, use proprietary technologies that are not readily modifiable when updates are needed, are subject to security vulnerabilities, and lack evidence of their effectiveness.[36]

Regulation typically draws on standard device approval and surveillance protocols by the FDA, but may be insufficient to address smart devices that contribute to clinical decision making. New machine learning applications possess natural language processing (NLP) algorithms that can capture natural spoken language and convert it to text, then further categorize the text data. Coupled with artificial intelligence, applications have potential to predict disease states and outcomes, and make suggestions regarding evidence-based treatments. Traditional face-to-face encounters do not capture the entirety of data that are exchanged between patients and care providers; however, NLP provides this technical capability.

Price[37] suggests a new governance approach with FDA oversight that enables disclosure of algorithm content and iterative measurement of effectiveness via

> **Box 2**
> **Reframing telehealth: a to-do list**
>
> - Redefine telehealth to focus less on modality and more on connectivity of information
> - Implement new hybrid delivery models that blend traditional telehealth modalities with in-person care
> - Update legal and regulatory standards to align with currently available technology surrounding data accuracy, data exchange, privacy, and security
> - Focus legislation on adaptability to evolving clinical technology as opposed to parity with face-to-face care
> - Continue support of interstate license reform
> - Enable simultaneous care by multiple providers to multiple patients by reevaluating concepts of provider-to-patient relationships and existing health plan benefit restrictions
> - Promote ongoing efforts among clinicians to define the role of artificial intelligence and machine learning in care delivery
> - Support new regulatory initiatives to capture and analyze real-world data on device performance
> - Test and adopt payment models that reward outcomes, efficiency, and reduced cost in lieu of the sum of separate components of care
> - Identify and scale pilot programs that show favorable evidence for clinical use and cost

real-world data feedback, which would serve to protect patients as well as foster innovation. Additional standardization considerations for data transfer from medical devices, similar to those developed for medical imaging known as DICOM (Digital Imaging and Communication in Medicine) standards, would make adoption of data collected by remote monitoring devices more universally accepted.

The growth of technology enabling remote communication and monitoring also raises the question of whether telehealth is new care, apart and distinct from but mirroring traditional face-to-face care, or whether it serves as an adjunct to existing in-person services. These distinctions may dictate whether virtual care continues to follow regulatory and payment parameters set by in-person care. Several investigators propose that telehealth has great potential to better enable access, quality, patient experience, and cost mitigation by integrating remote services into existing face-to-face workflows.[28,38]

In contrast, telehealth as a separately administered and financed service has potential to further fragment care delivery if it establishes dual medical record systems, disrupts care coordination, or creates disparity by limiting care to segments of the population able to access the requisite communication technology.[8] Although promising, technical limitations continue to impede the ability to integrate documentation within respective platforms into existing enterprise electronic health record systems, because this integration consists of site-by-site integration that must be custom built to accommodate each site.

SUMMARY: BEYOND THE LIMITATIONS

Telehealth has been successfully implemented across a variety of medical specialties with positive results. There are multiple categories of telehealth solutions, including synchronous, asynchronous, telemonitoring, and hybrid models, that permit various pathways among health care providers and between patients and providers to exchange health data, and to diagnose and treat. Telehealth solutions also provide an efficient platform to deliver patient education, which can be crucial to mitigating disease.

Despite regulatory activity and policy development at federal, state, and local levels, silos continue to limit central coordination and communication among telehealth stakeholders. The existing paradigm of face-to-face care continues to affect innovative reimbursement and regulation of telehealth. Current regulation around privacy, security, and data transmission fails to meet the demands of the patient population for privacy and ownership of their own information, balanced with the full potential of data portability. Reimbursement driven by traditional fee-for-service models links telehealth to existing transactional workflows and volume-based reporting of encounters. In addition, evidence for appropriate use cases and cost scenarios remains specific to local health delivery and payment systems, and is largely unscaled because of regulatory and reimbursement variation outside these systems.

Stakeholders within telehealth are many, and include patients, clinicians, health systems, employers, payers, legislators, and innovators and providers of technology. The authors challenge all stakeholders to work creatively and stepwise to address barriers that prevent new methods of information exchange from becoming integral to everyday health care (**Box 2**). Realizing the potential of connected care relies on clinicians' ability to stretch beyond old definitions, rules, workflows, and payment models that were created in a world that preceded the current capabilities for data connectivity and communication technology.

DISCLOSURE

The authors have nothing to disclose.

REFERENCES

1. Tucson RV, Edmunds M, Hodgkins ML. Telehealth. N Engl J Med 2017;377(16): 1585–92. Available at: www.nejm.org. Accessed May 11, 2019.
2. Field MJ. Telemedicine: a guide to assessing telecommunications for health care. a guide to assessing telecommunications for health care | The National Academies Press. Available at: https://www.nap.edu/catalog/5296/telemedicine-a-guide-to-assessing-telecommunications-for-health-care. Accessed May 11, 2019.
3. Telemedicine: opportunities and developments in member states. Available at: https://www.who.int/goe/publications/goe_telemedicine_2010.pdf. Accessed May 11, 2019.
4. Kwong MW. State health laws & reimbursement policies. Center for Connected Health Policy; 2018. Available at: https://www.cchpca.org/. Accessed May 11, 2019.
5. Schoenfeld AJ, Sehgal NJ, Auerbach A. The challenges of mobile health regulation. JAMA Intern Med 2016;176(5):704.
6. Center for Devices and Radiological Health. National evaluation system for health technology (NEST). U.S. Food and Drug Administration. Available at: https://www.fda.gov/about-fda/cdrh-reports/national-evaluation-system-health-technology-nest. Accessed May 11, 2019.
7. Mandl KD, Kohane IS. Time for a patient-driven health information economy? N Engl J Med 2016;374(3):205–8.
8. Marshall M, Shah R, Stokes-Lampard H. Online consulting in general practice: making the move from disruptive innovation to mainstream service. BMJ 2018; 360:k1195.

9. Alaska state legislature. Available at: http://www.akleg.gov/PDF/29/Bills/SB0098C.PDF. Accessed May 11, 2019.

10. FTC response to SB 74 Alaska 2016 . FTC response to SB 74 Alaska 2016. Available at: https://www.ftc.gov/system/files/documents/advocacy_documents/ftc-staff-comment-alaska-state-legislature-regarding-telehealth-provisions-senate-bill-74-which/160328alaskatelehealthcomment.pdf. Accessed May 11, 2019.

11. Interstate Medical Licensure Compact. Available at: https://imlcc.org/. Accessed May 11, 2019.

12. Florida Legislature Passes New Telehealth Law. Blogs | Health Care Law Today | Foley & Lardner LLP. Available at: https://www.foley.com/en/insights/publications/2019/05/florida-legislature-passes-new-telehealth-law. Accessed May 11, 2019.

13. 50-state survey: Establishment of a patient-physician relationship via telemedicine. 2018. Available at: https://www.ama-assn.org/system/files/2018-10/ama-chart-telemedicine-patient-physician-relationship.pdf. Accessed May 11, 2019.

14. Mass Health All Provider Bulletin. MassHealth all provider Bulletin 281 2019. Available at: https://www.mass.gov/files/documents/2019/01/23/all-provider-bulletin-281.pdf. Accessed May 11, 2019.

15. The Good and the Bad of the New MassHealth Telemedicine Rule. The National Law Review. Available at: https://www.natlawreview.com/article/good-and-bad-new-masshealth-telemedicine-rule. Accessed May 11, 2019.

16. Ethical Practice in Telemedicine. American Medical Association. Available at: https://www.ama-assn.org/delivering-care/ethics/ethical-practice-telemedicine. Accessed May 11, 2019.

17. Daniel H, Sulmasy LS. Policy recommendations to guide the use of telemedicine in primary care settings: an American College of Physicians Position Paper. Ann Intern Med 2015;163(10):787.

18. Practice Management Center. Teledermatology | American Academy of Dermatology. Available at: https://www.aad.org/practicecenter/managing-a-practice/teledermatology. Accessed May 11, 2019.

19. Moore MA, Coffman M, Jetty A, et al. Graham Center Policy One-Pager: Only 15% of FPs Report Using Telehealth; Training and Lack of Reimbursement Are Top Barriers. Am Fam Physician 2016;15(93):101. Available at: https://www.aafp.org/afp/2016/0115/p101.html.

20. Ackerman B. Is the Doctor In? Medical Malpractice Issues in the Age of Telemedicine. [online] The National Law Review. 2019. Available at: https://www.natlawreview.com/article/doctor-medical-malpractice-issues-age-telemedicine. Accessed June 19, 2019.

21. Legacy.americantelemed.org. (2019). State Telemedicine Gaps Reports - ATA Main. [online]. Available at: https://legacy.americantelemed.org/policy-page/state-telemedicine-gaps-reports. Accessed May 11, 2019.

22. Cms.gov. Medicare Physician Fee Schedule. 2019. Available at: https://www.cms.gov/Outreach-and-Education/Medicare-Learning-Network-MLN/MLNProducts/downloads/MedcrePhysFeeSchedfctsht.pdf. Accessed June 19, 2019.

23. Cms.gov. 2019. Available at: https://www.cms.gov/Outreach-and-Education/Medicare-Learning-Network-MLN/MLNMattersArticles/Downloads/MM11063.pdf. Accessed May 11, 2019.

24. Nussbaum S, McClellan M, Conway P. Paying Providers For Value: The Path Forward (Update) | Health Affairs. [online] Healthaffairs.org. 2019. Available at: https://www.healthaffairs.org/do/10.1377/hblog20160114.052635/full/. Accessed May 11, 2019.

25. Innovation.cms.gov. 2019. Available at: https://innovation.cms.gov/Files/reports/rtc-2018.pdf?utm_source=MC_NL_19-04-26_gen_vers-B&utm_campaign=MC_NL_2019-04-26&utm_medium=email. Accessed 11 May 2019.

26. Effectivehealthcare.ahrq.gov. Telehealth: mapping the evidence for patient outcomes from systematic reviews. 2019. Available at: https://effectivehealthcare.ahrq.gov/sites/default/files/pdf/telehealth_technical-brief.pdf. Accessed June 19, 2019.

27. Sousa C, Leite S, Lagido R, et al. Telemonitoring in heart failure: a state-of-the-art review. Rev Port Cardiol 2014;33(4):229–39.

28. Fraiche AM, Eapen ZJ, Mcclellan MB. Moving beyond the walls of the clinic. JACC Heart Fail 2017;5(4):297–304.

29. Telehealth. [online]. 2019. Available at: Pcori.org; https://www.pcori.org/research-results/topics/telehealth. Accessed June 19, 2019.

30. Mahar J, Rosencrance G, Rasmussen P. Telemedicine: Past, present, and future. Cleve Clin J Med 2018;85(12):938–42.

31. Ashwood JS, Mehrotra A, Cowling D, et al. Direct-to-consumer telehealth may increase access to care but does not decrease spending. Health Aff 2017;36(3):485–91.

32. Anderson D, Villagra V, Coman EN, et al. A cost-effectiveness analysis of cardiology eConsults for Medicaid patients. AJMC; 2018. Available at: https://www.ajmc.com/journals/issue/2018/2018-vol24-n1/a-costeffectiveness-analysis-of-cardiology-econsults-for-medicaid-patients. Accessed May 11, 2019.

33. VA Telehealth Services. VA Telehealth Services. VA Telehealth Services Home. 2013. Available at: https://www.telehealth.va.gov/. Accessed May 11, 2019.

34. Kane CK, Gillis K. The use of telemedicine by physicians: still the exception rather than the rule. Health Affairs. 2018. Available at: https://www.healthaffairs.org/doi/10.1377/hlthaff.2018.05077. Accessed May 11, 2019.

35. Denicola NG, Lowery CL, Marko KI, et al. A Systematic review of telehealth on clinical outcomes in obstetrics & gynecology [27E]. Obstet Gynecol 2019;133:585S[JM1].

36. Ho A, Quick O. Leaving patients to their own devices? Smart technology, safety and therapeutic relationships. BMC Med Ethics 2018;19(18):1–6. Available at: https://bmcmedethics.biomedcentral.com/articles/10.1186/s12910-018-0255-8. Accessed May 11, 2019.

37. Price WN. Regulating Black-Box Medicine. Michigan Law Review. Available at: https://michiganlawreview.org/regulating-black-box-medicine/. Accessed June 19, 2019.

38. Lerouge C, Garfield M. Crossing the telemedicine chasm: have the U.S. barriers to widespread adoption of telemedicine been significantly reduced? Int J Environ Res Public Health 2013;10(12):6472–84.

Telemedicine in Low-Risk Obstetrics

Julie R. Whittington, MD*, Abigail M. Ramseyer, DO, Chad B. Taylor, MD

KEYWORDS

- Telemedicine • Obstetrics • Virtual prenatal care • Gestational weight gain
- Smoking cessation • Rural obstetric care

KEY POINTS

- Pregnant women living in rural communities face several barriers to prenatal care, including limited access to local perinatal care, long travel times to receive care, increased stress due to the limitations, and increased maternal and neonatal morbidity and mortality.
- Telemedicine has been utilized to extend specialty prenatal care to rural patients. This service may be applied to routine prenatal care as well to serve those living in maternity care deserts.
- Telemedicine has application in prenatal and postnatal care.
- Implemented telemedicine programs have excellent provider and patient satisfaction, reduce travel time and time away from work for patients, improve the access to and quality of care, and support isolated providers.

INTRODUCTION

Telemedicine has been used in perinatal care for several years but has focused mostly in the capacity of specialty care.[1–3] Examples of use in obstetrics include genetic counseling, maternal-fetal medicine subspecialty consultation, interpretation of ultrasounds and nonstress tests, and management of diabetes and postpartum depression.[1,3] The principles of telemedicine may be expanded to routine obstetric care and may provide an improvement to the diminishing access rural women have to perinatal services and quality of care, while also supporting rural providers. Subsequently, this may assist with improvements in maternal and neonatal outcomes. Telemedicine may be of particular benefit for routine prenatal and postpartum care in areas where resources are limited. Expansion of remote monitoring may reduce the travel and financial burdens for pregnant women by reducing the number of in-office visits. Expanding remote visits can reduce stress and lead to improved patient satisfaction with their prenatal care. Programs also have implemented behavioral modification tools to encourage tobacco cessation and to monitor and limit weight gain in

University of Medical Sciences, Department of Obstetrics and Gynecology, 4301 West Markham Street, Slot 518, Little Rock, AR 72205, USA
* Corresponding author.
E-mail address: jrwhittington@uams.edu

Obstet Gynecol Clin N Am 47 (2020) 241–247
https://doi.org/10.1016/j.ogc.2020.02.006
0889-8545/20/Published by Elsevier Inc.

pregnancy. This article outlines applications of telemedicine in providing routine obstetrics care in the prenatal and postnatal periods and how it can support rural providers and provides commentary on provider and patient satisfaction with current programs.

TELEMEDICINE, PRENATAL VISIT REDUCTION, AND PATIENT SATISFACTION

As the physician shortage across the United States spreads, finding ways to decrease the workload without compromising maternal and fetal care is a paramount goal.[4] Reducing obstetric visits by alternating telemedicine visits with advanced practice nurses with physician visits is one way to accomplish this. One large prospective study examined a reduction from 14 patient visits to 9 visits with interspersed virtual advanced practice nurse visits.[5] They found no significantly increased risks to mother or baby. The investigators concluded that this model of care likely can free time in provider schedules to focus on other patients. They noted that they did not perform a cost analysis of this practice.[5] In this study, patients were instructed to measure their own blood pressures and use a handheld fetal Doppler. The ease of connecting for the visits and the quality of connection were complicating factors, indicating that videoconference platform selection may play a key role in overall patient satisfaction, including familiarity and comfort with the applications (apps).[5]

Another prospective study used registered nurse virtual visits alternating with nurse-midwife and physician visits.[6] In this study, patients appreciated the continuity the visits provided with their nurses and felt empowered by the knowledge provided by obtaining their own data. One important caveat to this study is that a majority of these patients were white, married, privately insured, and highly educated: this population traditionally has had better obstetric outcomes than minority, single, low socioeconomic status patients.

There is an obvious concern that reduction in traditional face-to-face visits may lead to decreased patient satisfaction. In 2017, a randomized trial of 430 virtual care patients receiving at least some of their prenatal care via virtual visit maintained that a mixed model of care was found to have significantly higher satisfaction rates compared with traditional care.[1] In a 2019 randomized controlled trial of 300 women, women were randomized to the reduced prenatal visit model with virtual visits or usual care. In the reduced visit model, there were 8 onsite appointments and 6 virtual visits. The researchers found that the reduced visit model saved 2.8 obstetric appointments per patient. The patients in the virtual care group notably had significantly increased patient satisfaction and lower pregnancy-related stress.[7]

TELEMEDICINE AND BEHAVIORAL MODIFICATION

Telemedicine also can be used to assist with modification of obstetric risk factors. Cell phone apps have been used to mitigate weight gain and decrease cigarette smoking in pregnancy and the preconception period. As society is increasingly reliant on technology, women who are pregnant frequently use the Internet and cell phone apps for information.[8] Steegers[9] introduced a mobile health (mHealth) platform to reach periconceptional patients on the topics of poor nutritional status, smoking, and obesity. Van Dijk and colleagues[10] used an mHealth system to alert patients of their risk and gave incentives for behavioral changes. Usage of the app was high, with 65% of participants completing the coaching. Foster and colleagues[11] completed a pilot study that looked at an mHealth app to promote pregnancy, postpartum, and interconception health; 14 women participated in the study, and they learned that in the interconception period, women were less likely to engage with the system. Preconception intervention is ideal because this establishes a foundation for a healthy pregnancy.

Before pregnancy is undertaken and after a patient delivers, contraception is important for optimizing patient care. One way to increase access to contraception is through telecontraception. A study in 2019 was performed to evaluate the safety of such encounters. Secret shoppers were utilized to serve as standardized patients with a variety of relative and absolute contraindications. Adherence to the Centers for Disease Control and Prevention Medical Eligibility Criteria for Contraceptive Use was 93%; the average visit time was 7.5 minutes. This convenience combined with safety is likely appealing to patients; however, it also was noted that most companies offering these services did not counsel patients about long-acting reversible contraception, a more effective choice for many patients.[12]

Once pregnancy has been established, mHealth apps also have been used to encourage smoking cessation and assess patient risk. Leavitt and colleagues[13] used Text4baby to recruit pregnant smokers to enroll patients in Quit4baby and noted patients responded best to emotional appeals to personal pride. They also showed that text messages can be effective for recruiting study participants, which can be important for future research. The effectiveness of this intervention for smoking cessation has not yet been established; however. Krishnamurti and colleagues[14] used the myHealthyPregnancy app to assess patient risks for preterm birth and communicate those risks to patients. Women who participated had much higher attendance at prenatal appointments than baseline attendance; their intention to breastfeed increased; and they qualitatively expressed appreciation for risk feedback in the pregnancy.

TELEMEDICINE AND GESTATIONAL WEIGHT GAIN

Gestational weight gain is associated with adverse perinatal outcomes, such as diabetes, gestational hypertension, and obesity. In a 2015 study, text messages along with diet and activity goal setting were used to minimize gestational weight gain in obese patients.[15] The investigators found a decreased mean gestational weight gain in the intervention group compared with usual care; however, this study is limited by small sample size. Graham and colleagues[16] used an electronic health intervention to reduce the risk of excess weight gain in pregnancy in a randomized controlled trial. In the intervention arm, participants used a weight gain tracker along with diet and physical activity tools. In the other arm, the patients simply had access to a Web site with blogs, articles, and frequently asked questions. Consistent users of their intervention gained less weight when adjusted for socioeconomic status and body mass index. Good nutrition and a healthy lifestyle are known to benefit pregnancy outcomes. Further apps are being developed to bring reliable nutrition counseling to pregnant patients.[17] One prospective study of online interventions in gestational weight gain found no difference in the intervention group compared with the control group; however, the researchers noted low utilization of the behavioral tools.[18]

A recent randomized controlled trial compared mHealth technology interventions in overweight pregnant women (body mass index >25 kg/m^2) to routine obstetric care. The primary outcome in this study was incidence of gestational diabetes, whereas secondary outcomes include gestational weight gain and maternal activity level. There were no differences in the primary or secondary outcomes in the 2 groups.[19]

More research needs to be done to establish the effectiveness of online interventions on gestational weight gain; however, preliminary data seem to show benefits from telehealth interventions when patients increase utilization of the programs.

RURAL PERINATAL CARE: BARRIERS TO AND APPLICATION OF TELEMEDICINE

Approximately 18 million reproductive age women live in rural communities in the United States, with approximately 500,000 births annually. Medicaid is the largest payer of perinatal care, with a higher proportion of coverage in rural communities. In 2016, Medicaid funded 43% of all births in the United States. The Centers for Medicare & Medicaid Services (CMS) published its first "Rural Health Strategy" in 2018, focusing on improving maternal health care in the rural setting, especially in light of the national movement to decrease maternal mortality and severe maternal morbidity while improving neonatal outcomes.[20] It is well established that access to quality perinatal care is crucial for maintaining maternal health and positive neonatal outcomes. Broadly, access to perinatal care may be defined by "availability of hospitals providing obstetric care, availability of providers offering obstetric care and access to that care through health insurance."[21]

Rural communities have seen significant economic effects from the modern-era Great Recession and have not seen a comparable amount of recovery as seen in metropolitan and urban counties. Rural communities see 200,000 lost jobs annually, resulting in increasing unemployment rates. In most rural communities, the hospital system is the largest or second largest employer, making it integral to the economic infrastructure of the community. Closure of small, local hospitals has a significant impact on the economy, unemployment rates, and overall health of the community because access to care is lost. Between 2010 and 2018, 83 rural hospitals have closed and 674 are vulnerable to closure due mostly to operation for loss; "44% of rural hospitals operate at a loss and 30% operate below a -3% margin." In 2018, an infrastructure plan was introduced to provide federal funding to support and modernize rural communities devoid of resources.[22]

Maternal health care has been impacted by the economic climate with 179 rural counties losing or closing their obstetric services between 2004 and 2014, correlating to a 9% loss, and leaving only 49% of rural women with access to perinatal services within a 30-minute drive[20,23–25]; 10% of rural women are now forced to drive 100 or more miles to receive prenatal care. This affects not only intrapartum care but also prenatal and postpartum care.[20] Increased travel requirements also place a burden on pregnant patients. Anxiety regarding reaching a hospital in time for delivery increases psychological stress for patients. The costs of travel and time out of work place financial stressors on pregnant women and their families, especially patients who live significant distances from obstetric care, who frequently relocate at approximately 36 weeks' gestation in preparation for childbirth.[26] Common reasons for closing obstetric units include low volume of deliveries, difficulties in maintaining appropriate staffing, safety concerns, and a high percentage of Medicaid-funded patients, which may leave hospitals financially vulnerable.[27]

Closure of obstetric services has created maternity care deserts, which are defined as counties "in which access to maternity health care services is limited or absent, either through lack of services or barriers to a woman's ability to access that care."[21] As of 2018, 1085 counties have been deemed maternal care deserts, with more than 5 million women residing in these counties without a hospital that offers obstetric services; 150,000 babies are born annually to women of maternal desert counties and an additional 10 million women live in counties with limited perinatal care.[21] Lack of access to maternal health care has significant negative impact on perinatal outcomes, including higher rates of preterm birth, low birth weight infants, maternal mortality, severe maternal morbidiity, and postpartum depression. Women living in rural communities are more likely to present for prenatal care late in pregnancy.[20] Lack of education, lower health literacy, unintended pregnancy, lack of health insurance coverage, and poor transportation all have been implicated as confounding factors.[20] Rural hospitals also report higher rates of adverse obstetric outcomes, such as postpartum hemorrhage and blood transfusion.[23] A retrospective cohort study published in 2018 analyzed approximately 5 million births and found that loss of obstetric services in counties not adjacent to urban areas was associated with more out-of-hospital births, preterm deliveries, and deliveries in hospitals without obstetric services.[24]

Perinatal care providers include obstetrician-gynecologists, certified nurse-midwives/certified midwives, and family medicine physicians. Additionally, nurse practitioners assist with providing antepartum and postpartum care.[21] Many rural communities rely on general surgeons to perform cesarean deliveries.[28] Family medicine physicians, who historically have provided a majority of prenatal and obstetric in rural areas, are performing fewer deliveries and providing less prenatal care.[28] Reported reasons for the cessation of practicing obstetrics by family medicine physicians and obstetricians-gynecologists include malpractice concerns in the current litigation climate, exhaustion, desire for work-life balance, adverse outcomes, lack of hospital support or infrastructure, stressors of being a sole provider, decreased reimbursement, and high malpractice insurance costs.[25,29] Additionally, family medicine physicians report insufficient training; inadequate numbers of patients to maintain skills; lack of hospital support in regard to privileges; lack of clinical support; lack of other specialties', subspecialties', and obstetricians'/gynecologists' back-up support; and institutional political concerns, including discouragement from practicing obstetrics, as contributors to no longer offering perinatal care services.[29] Telemedicine has the capacity to assist with saving rural providers and developing a workforce as well and is a concept supported by CMS.[20]

Programs have been started that combine home visits with face-to-face in-office visits to provide prenatal care to rural women. Benefits of this include decreased financial travel burdens, high patient satisfaction, and empowerment of women to be invested in their own care.[1,20] Offering postpartum home virtual visits may improve completion of the postpartum visit, allow for breastfeeding support, and improve screening and detecting of postpartum depression, which may lead to improved treatment of postpartum depression and establishment of a contraception plan.

Telemedicine also is useful for supporting rural providers. The University of Arkansas for Medical Sciences (UAMS) launched a statewide initiative to educate emergency departments and labor and delivery units and provide a hypertension bundle for management of hypertensive emergencies in pregnancy and the postpartum period. The UAMS Institute for Digital Health & Innovation High Risk Pregnancy Program (formerly ANGELS) is another example of distant support to rural providers. This program was established to increase access to and improve perinatal services around the state.[2,20] The High Risk Pregnancy Program provides a Web site with guidelines for routine and complicated obstetric and neonatal topics, a 24-hour call center for provider and patient support, 24-hour access to maternal-fetal medicine consultation, and education to improve rural providers' readiness to manage obstetric emergencies.[2] A recent survey of High Risk Pregnancy Program patients noted a 98.8% satisfaction rate, and 95% indicated they would use it in the future. In this same study, providers who utilized the service noted increased access to health care (97.1%), improvements in the lives of patients (92.5%), and that the telehealth system is "excellent" (98.5%).[30]

SUMMARY

Telemedicine has expanding uses in routine obstetric care and can be used to extend the reach of obstetricians to maternity care deserts. It also can help contribute to maternal safety and satisfaction both during the pregnancy and postpartum. There are many forms of telemedicine, from provider visits to electronic health apps. More research should be done on ways to increase the efficacy of electronic health interventions.

DISCLOSURE

The authors have no commercial or financial conflicts of interest.

REFERENCES

1. Pflugeisen BM, Mou J. Patient satisfaction with virtual obstetric care. Matern Child Health J 2017;21(7):1544–51.
2. Lowery C, Bronstein J, McGhee J, et al. ANGELS and University of Arkansas for Medical Sciences paradigm for distant obstetrical care delivery. Am J Obstet Gynecol 2007;196(6):534.e1–9.
3. Magann EF, McKelvey SS, Hitt WC, et al. The use of telemedicine in obstetrics: a review of the literature. Obstet Gynecol Surv 2011;66(3):170–8.
4. Rosenberg J. Physician shortage likely to impact OB/GYN workforce in coming years secondary physician shortage likely to impact OB/GYN workforce in coming years. 2019. Available at: https://www.ajmc.com/newsroom/physician-shortage-likely-to-impact-obgyn-workforce-in-coming-years.
5. Pflugeisen BM, McCarren C, Poore S, et al. Virtual visits: managing prenatal care with modern technology. MCN Am J Matern Child Nurs 2016;41(1):24–30.
6. Baron AM, Ridgeway JL, Stirn SL, et al. Increasing the connectivity and autonomy of RNs with low-risk obstetric patients. Am J Nurs 2018;118(1):48–55.
7. Butler Tobah YS, LeBlanc A, Branda ME, et al. Randomized comparison of a reduced-visit prenatal care model enhanced with remote monitoring. Am J Obstet Gynecol 2019;221(6):638.e1–8.
8. Wallwiener S, Muller M, Doster A, et al. Pregnancy eHealth and mHealth: user proportions and characteristics of pregnant women using Web-based information sources-a cross-sectional study. Arch Gynecol Obstet 2016;294(5):937–44.
9. Steegers-Theunissen RPM. Periconception mHealth platform for prevention of placental-related outcomes and non-communicable diseases. Placenta 2017; 60:115–8.
10. Van Dijk MR, Huijgen NA, Willemsen SP, et al. Impact of an mHealth platform for pregnancy on nutrition and lifestyle of the reproductive population: a survey. JMIR mHealth uHealth 2016;4(2):e53.
11. Foster J, Miller L, Isbell S, et al. mHealth to promote pregnancy and interconception health among African-American women at risk for adverse birth outcomes: a pilot study. mHealth 2015;1:20.
12. Jain T, Schwarz EB, Mehrotra A. A Study of Telecontraception. N Engl J Med 2019;381(13):1287–8.
13. Leavitt L, Abroms L, Johnson P, et al. Recruiting pregnant smokers from Text4-baby for a randomized controlled trial of Quit4baby. Transl Behav Med 2017; 7(2):157–65.

14. Krishnamurti T, Davis AL, Wong-Parodi G, et al. Development and testing of the myhealthypregnancy app: a behavioral decision research-based tool for assessing and communicating pregnancy risk. JMIR mHealth uHealth 2017;5(4):e42.
15. Soltani H, Duxbury AM, Arden MA, et al. Maternal obesity management using mobile technology: a feasibility study to evaluate a text messaging based complex intervention during pregnancy. J Obes 2015;2015:814830.
16. Graham ML, Strawderman MS, Demment M, et al. Does usage of an ehealth intervention reduce the risk of excessive gestational weight gain? secondary analysis from a randomized controlled trial. J Med Internet Res 2017;19(1):e6.
17. Johnsen H, Blom KF, Lee A, et al. Using eHealth to increase autonomy supportive care: a multicenter intervention study in antenatal care. Comput Inform Nurs 2018;36(2):77–83.
18. Olson CM, Groth SW, Graham ML, et al. The effectiveness of an online intervention in preventing excessive gestational weight gain: the e-moms roc randomized controlled trial. BMC Pregnancy Childbirth 2018;18(1):148.
19. Kennelly MA, Ainscough K, Lindsay KL, et al. Pregnancy exercise and nutrition with smartphone application support: a randomized controlled trial. Obstet Gynecol 2018;131(5):818–26.
20. Services CfMaM. Improving access to maternal health care in rural communities issue brief. Secondary improving access to maternal health care in rural communities issue brief 09/03/2019. 2019. Available at: https://www.cms.gov/About-CMS/Agency-Information/OMH/equity-initiatives/rural-health/09032019-Maternal-Health-Care-in-Rural-Communities.pdf.
21. Nowhere to go: maternity care deserts across the U.S. Secondary Nowhere to go: maternity care deserts across the U.S. 2018. Available at: https://www.marchofdimes.org/materials/Nowhere_to_Go_Final.pdf.
22. Seigel J. Rebuild Rural: The Importance of health Care in Infrastructure. Rural Health Voices 2018 2/20/2018. Available at: https://www.ruralhealthweb.org/blogs/ruralhealthvoices/february-2018/rebuild-rural-the-importance-of-health-care-in-in. Accessed December 1, 2019.
23. Hung P, Henning-Smith CE, Casey MM, et al. Access to obstetric services in rural counties still declining, with 9 percent losing services, 2004-14. Health Aff (Millwood) 2017;36(9):1663–71.
24. Kozhimannil KB, Hung P, Henning-Smith C, et al. Association between loss of hospital-based obstetric services and birth outcomes in rural counties in the United States. JAMA 2018;319(12):1239–47.
25. ACOG Committee Opinion No. 586: Health disparities in rural women. Obstet Gynecol 2014;123(2 Pt 1):384–8.
26. Grzybowski S, Stoll K, Kornelsen J. Distance matters: a population based study examining access to maternity services for rural women. BMC Health Serv Res 2011;11:147.
27. Hung P, Kozhimannil KB, Casey MM, et al. Why are obstetric units in rural hospitals closing their doors? Health Serv Res 2016;51(4):1546–60.
28. Kozhimannil KB, Casey MM, Hung P, et al. The rural obstetric workforce in us hospitals: challenges and opportunities. J Rural Health 2015;31(4):365–72.
29. Avery DM, McDonald JT Jr. The declining number of family physicians practicing obstetrics: rural impact, reasons, recommendations and considerations. American Journal of Clinical Medicine 2014;10(2):70–8.
30. Bhandari NR, Payakachat N, Fletcher DA, et al. Validation of newly developed surveys to evaluate patients' and providers' satisfaction with telehealth obstetric services. Telemed J E Health 2019. https://doi.org/10.1089/tmj.2019.0156.

Telemedicine in High-Risk Obstetrics

Julie R. Whittington, MD[a],*, Everett F. Magann, MD[b]

KEYWORDS

- Telemedicine • Teleultrasound • High-risk obstetrics • Diabetes in pregnancy
- Hypertension in pregnancy

KEY POINTS

- Telemedicine is well accepted by both patients and their providers.
- Telemedicine is used in the management of diabetes, hypertension, and other high-risk conditions in at-risk pregnancies and for the detection of fetal anomalies at the time of a patient's targeted ultrasounds.
- Telemedicine has the ability to quickly increase access to care.
- Uses for telemedicine continue to change and expand.

INTRODUCTION

Telemedicine is the use of telecommunications and technology to diagnose, counsel, and treat patients from a remote site. It also has been defined as the use of technology to assist in the sharing of medical information and provision of services between providers and patients.[1] Telemedicine has been used to treat high-risk pregnancy conditions, such as diabetes mellitus and hypertension; it also has been used to screen for and treat postpartum depression.[2] Telemedicine is used during sonographic screening for fetal anomalies and has been shown to be as accurate as on-site ultrasound.[3] A Belgian study showed the cost-effectiveness of home monitoring systems and remote surveillance for bleeding in pregnancy, preterm labor, hypertension, fetal abnormalities, placental abnormalities, and polyhydramnios.[4]

The applications of telemedicine in high-risk obstetrics are promising means of reducing the cost burden of high-quality maternity care. High-risk obstetric services in medically underserved areas are needed to improve access to maternity care. In the United States, 700 women die each year due to a pregnancy-related cause.[5] Telemedicine is specifically cited by a maternal mortality review committee in 2019 as a means for

[a] University of Arkansas for Medical Sciences, 4301 West Markham Street, Slot 518, Little Rock, AR 72205, USA; [b] Department of OB/GYN, MFM Division, 4301 West Markham Street, Slot 518, Little Rock, AR 72205, USA
* Corresponding author.
E-mail address: jrwhittington@uams.edu

Obstet Gynecol Clin N Am 47 (2020) 249–257
https://doi.org/10.1016/j.ogc.2020.02.007
0889-8545/20/Published by Elsevier Inc.

facilities without obstetric providers to obtain appropriate consultative care for their patients.[6] Thus, telemedicine may have an important role in reducing maternal mortality.

TELEMEDICINE AND HYPERTENSIVE DISORDERS OF PREGNANCY

Hypertensive disorders of pregnancy affect 2% to 8% of pregnancies worldwide and are a leading cause of maternal mortality in both developing and developed countries.[7] Hypertensive disorders are a continuum and include the diagnoses of gestational hypertension, preeclampsia (with or without severe features), chronic hypertension with superimposed preeclampsia, and eclampsia. Prompt diagnosis and treatment mitigate the maternal risks associated with preeclampsia. Telemedicine is utilized to triage patient symptoms, to remotely monitor blood pressure in the antepartum and postpartum periods, and for the management of preeclampsia.

Ambulatory blood pressure monitoring in pregnant patients has been used to identify women at risk for preeclampsia. Ganapathy and colleagues[8] used a kit with a Bluetooth-enabled blood pressure machine and an Android-based mobile phone to surveil and triage hypertensive patients. This kit reduced patient visits, and more than 90% of patients found it simple to use. Lanssens and colleagues[9] performed a 2-year retrospective study comparing their remote monitoring program with conventional care. Remote monitoring included a wireless blood pressure monitor, a weight scale, and an activity tracker. The data were transmitted to an online dashboard staffed by a midwife, and further assessment was triggered for weight gain greater than 1 kg/d and if blood pressure was greater than 140 mm Hg systolic or greater than 90 mm Hg diastolic. This remote monitoring program reduced the total number of prenatal visits, decreased the prevalence of preeclampsia, and allowed for women to labor spontaneously more frequently than women in the conventional care group. A follow-up study reviewed and confirmed the cost benefit of remote monitoring compared with conventional care. A follow-up study of the same group found a 50% cost reduction with the remote monitoring group. A reduction in the neonatal hospital stay drove the majority of the cost savings, because patients at less than 34 weeks' gestation in the remote monitoring group had an average of 10 days of pregnancy prolongation compared with the conventional care group.[10]

Mobile health (mHealth) applications extend the reach of health care providers and improve patient access to care. Dunsmuir and colleagues[11] developed a protocol using a Phone Oximeter, patient symptoms, and blood pressure with a decision tree to assist nurses and midwives with patient care. This mHealth application specifically offers guidance on when to give magnesium sulfate, treat with antihypertensives, and proceed with delivery, leading to timely intervention in low-income to middle-income settings.

The postpartum period is characterized by fluid shifts and increases in blood pressure, especially in postpartum days 3 to 5. Hoppe and colleagues[12] studied home monitoring of blood pressures with transmission of data daily and telehealth visits 48 hours after discharge. Participants received tablets, blood pressure cuffs, weight scales, and oxygen sensors that synced with a central monitoring platform. In this group of women, 45% required an increase in blood pressure medication or the initiation of blood pressure medication. No patients required readmission, and 87% of women were very satisfied with their remote monitoring. Rhoads and colleagues[13] investigated implementation of mHealth technology in 48 postpartum women with a hypertension diagnosis on hospital discharge. They found women were comfortable with mHealth usage and that text messages were the preferred method for the health care providers to contact them.

Telemedicine appears to be a promising technology to enhance the surveillance of women in an ambulatory setting with hypertensive disorders of pregnancy. More studies are needed, however, to determine if telehealth applications reduce maternal and/or neonatal morbidity and mortality.

TELEMEDICINE AND DIABETES MELLITUS IN PREGNANCY

Pregestational diabetes mellitus and gestational diabetes mellitus (GDM) both are defined by maternal hyperglycemia, which has effects on the mother, the placenta, and the fetus. Pregestational diabetes affects 2.2% of all pregnancies in the United States and GDM may affect up to 9.2% of all pregnancies in the United States.[14,15] As the percentage of women entering pregnancy who are either overweight or obese surges, there are likely to be further escalations in both pregestational diabetes mellitus and GDM. Complications associated with diabetes in pregnancy include intrauterine fetal demise, fetal macrosomia, increased incidence of cesarean delivery, and increased risk of hypertensive disorders of pregnancy.

Telemedicine assists with maternal glucose control through the transfer of data and advice between providers and patients. The goal of glucose control is reduction in the rates of adverse pregnancy outcomes associated with diabetes. Optimal management of diabetes mellitus requires frequent and timely assessment of maternal blood glucose values. Mackillop and colleagues[16] used an Android phone with a Bluetooth-linked glucometer with transmission to a Web site, which allowed for clinician review of results and medication adjustment within 24 hours to 72 hours. Women in this study were highly compliant, with 85% of women submitting at least 18 readings per week; unfortunately, pregnancy outcomes were not reported. Harrison and colleagues[17] looked at the acceptability of virtual prenatal visits for 10 women with GDM. They found telemedicine was highly acceptable to potential participants. The patients cited multiple benefits, including less time away from work, reducing childcare needs associated with visits, and learning self-management skills.

Ferrera and colleague18 used an integrated health delivery system with telehealth interventions to improve outcomes with GDM. Specifically, women in centers with consistent referrals to telephonic nurse management had decreased risk of delivering a macrosomic infant along with an increase in postpartum glucose testing.[18] Rasekaba and colleagues[19] utilized the Telemedicine for Gestational Diabetes Mellitus program, which involved accessible Web-based technology in addition to usual care. Diabetic nurse educators reviewed glucoses as frequently as every 2 days and assisted with titration of insulin in-between visits. Participants in the telemedicine group reached glycemic control 3 weeks faster (on average) than the usual care group though there was no difference between macrosomia, route of delivery, admission to special care nursery, or large-for-gestational-age infants between the groups. Nutrition interventions also been have utilized to assist with control of GDM. Yang and colleagues[20] used the WeChat platform, which included nutrition teaching, exercise instruction, and recording of blood glucoses. Their interventions led to decreased fasting blood glucose and 2-hour postprandial glucose levels, yet there was no difference in 1-hour postprandial glucose levels.

Many studies have been done on use of telemedicine technology and Internet-based self-monitoring. A systematic review and meta-analysis involving 832 patients looked at Internet-based self-monitoring programs compared with usual care and showed a decreased maternal hemoglobin A_{1C} (HbA_{1c}) and a decreased cesarean delivery rate.[21] Another systematic review and meta-analysis by Ming and colleagues[22] showed improvement in HbA_{1c} with telemedicine technologies but did not show any differences in maternal or neonatal outcomes. The benefit of telemedicine in the care of diabetes in pregnancy may be in decreased cesarean delivery rate, decreased patient visits, decreased costs, and increased ability to expand care overall, especially to underserved areas.

Finally, women with GDM have a 50% risk of developing type 2 diabetes mellitus in the future. Screening for prediabetes and type 2 diabetes mellitus is recommended in the postpartum period. Patient compliance with postpartum glucose testing, however, has been variable. Van Ryswyk and colleagues[23] sought to use text messaging reminders to patients with GDM at 6 weeks postpartum, 3 months postpartum, and 6 months postpartum compared with a single reminder at 12 weeks to 16 weeks postpartum. There were no differences between groups in the women who undertook postpartum glucose testing; nonetheless, both groups had very high compliance rates (77.6% and 76.8%, respectively). This may be because both groups received reminders and were enrolled in the study, which heightened awareness of the risks of subsequently developing diabetes.

TELEULTRASOUND AND SCREENING FOR FETAL ANOMALIES

Second-trimester ultrasound should be offered to all pregnant patients to screen for fetal anomalies as part of standard prenatal care.[24] Fetal teleultrasound offers the benefit of specialty consultation and review of images without a patient having to travel to a tertiary center. The first use of fetal telemedicine was described in 1996 by Fisk and colleagues.[25] They performed 39 teleconsultations and found image quality to be sufficient in all but 1 study. The women in the study felt that teleconsultation reduced their anxiety. In 2000, 24 24 teleultrasound consultations were carried out by Chan and colleagues,[26] with real-time transmission of ultrasound. They found teleultrasound to be technically feasible and accepted by clinicians and patients.

On a larger scale, the University of Arkansas for Medical Sciences Antenatal and Neonatal Guidelines, Education and Learning System (ANGELS) has a telemedicine endeavor providing health care to high-risk pregnant patients throughout the state. In 2001, 1050 patients had teleultrasounds and the program rapidly expanded. By 2011, 1897 comprehensive teleultrasounds were performed at 18 sites.[27] Rabie and colleagues[3] performed a retrospective cohort study of 2368 teleultrasounds and found sensitivity and specificity of teleultrasound to be comparable with on-site ultrasound. They were able to complete the anatomic survey on the first ultrasound in 82% of patients. This finding supports the use of teleultrasound for patients in remote areas because teleultrasound performed as well as on-site ultrasound.

Prenatal cardiac evaluation with ultrasound is essential for the detection of congenital heart abnormalities. Prenatal diagnosis of congenital heart disease allows for coordination of care and delivery planning; neonates can have increased morbidity and mortality before transfer can be arranged to a tertiary care center. Mistry and Gariner[28] examined cost-effectiveness of universal telemedicine screening for congenital heart disease in the United Kingdom in 2013. They found that offering teleultrasound screening to all standard-risk woman would be cost-effective, using a unique decision model.[28] Brown and Holland[29] successfully instituted a fetal tele-echocardiography program in rural Kentucky. Fetal tele-echo was accurate in identification of complex congenital heart disease and none of the patients with normal fetal tele-echocardiograms required higher levels of care.[29]

Teleultrasound and tele-echocardiography are acceptable to providers, have comparable sensitivity and specificity as on-site ultrasound, and may be cost-saving screening programs.

TELEMEDICINE AND OBSTETRIC SPECIALTY CONSULTATION FOR UNDERSERVED AREAS

Access to specialty care, lack of transportation, lack of appropriately trained personnel, care coordination, and timely consultation all are factors that can contribute to maternal morbidity and mortality.[6] The ANGELS is a state-wide program in Arkansas, which was founded in 2001, that has 5 elements to address these issues. These include a statewide telemedicine network, education and support for obstetric providers, case management services, a 24-hour call center, and an evidence-based guidelines development and distribution network.[30] In the first year after implementation, telemedicine consultations doubled and physician phone consultations doubled.[31] Bronstein and colleagues[32] found that between 2001 and 2006 that there was a shift toward referrals for appropriate diagnoses and a shift away from referrals without diagnoses recommended for consultation. In that same time period, maternal-fetal medicine telemedicine consultation increased from 7.6% to 13.3% of all consultative visits.[33] Ivey and colleagues[34] reviewed indications for telemedicine consults from rural counties in Arkansas where there were no obstetricians or limited obstetric services and observed that the most common indication for telemedicine consultation from 2011 to 2012 was diabetes mellitus. The investigators noted that telemedicine has the unique ability to provide maternal-fetal medicine consultations to women who would be unable to get specialty care otherwise due to lack of resources or a long distance from a specialist. Arkansas has telemedicine sites across the state to allow for patient access to specialty care (**Fig. 1**).

The 24-hour call center portion of ANGELS helps triage women and facilitate or expedite care if needed. Between 2004 and 2016, the call center handled 63,999 calls. The most commonly triaged complaint was preterm contractions. Reducing unnecessary labor and delivery visits is important for allocation of resources, which is of utmost importance in low-resource areas.[35] The ANGELS call center also serves to facilitate transfer from local hospitals to a higher-level of care, especially at premature gestational ages and for very-low-birth-weight (VLBW) infants.[36] After the implementation of ANGELS, transport of mothers with premature or VLBW infants tended to occur earlier and proactively.[37] Delivery of preterm infants in hospitals with appropriate levels of care is known to improve neonatal outcomes.

Obstetric telemedicine consults often involve counseling patients on diagnoses with poor perinatal prognosis. Wyatt and colleagues[38] 8 interviewed women 6 months to 24 months after delivery of their infants who had had poor prognosis about their telemedicine experience. A majority reported they would recommend friends and family for telemedicine consultation, even though they had received bad news. The patients also gave valuable advice for optimizing telemedicine consultation for future patients: recommendations included focusing the camera on 1 provider, limiting interruptions, establishing expectations, and giving feedback after the visit.[38] Telemedicine also is used by subspecialists from other disciplines to assist with prenatal care and counseling. Pediatric urologists used telemedicine to counsel patients on prognosis associated with teleultrasound-diagnosed fetal urologic disorders and plan location of delivery.[39] Telemedicine allows for care across distances and can be optimized for the best patient experiences.

OTHER MANAGEMENT ISSUES IN TELEMEDICINE IN HIGH-RISK OBSTETRICS

Telemedicine is used for a variety of other indications, including coordinating care for antepartum patients diagnosed with placenta accreta spectrum, medical decision making, monitoring preterm labor, and assessment for perinatal depression. In a

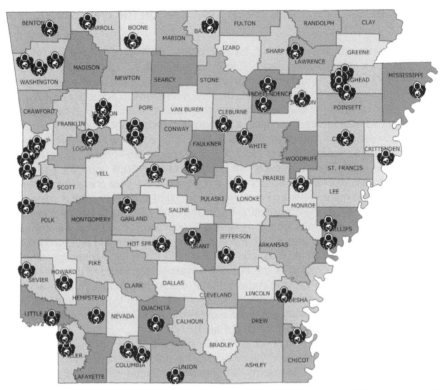

Fig. 1. The University of Arkansas for Medical Sciences ANGELS telemedicine program reaches across the state. (*Courtesy of* UAMS Institute for Digital Health & Innovation OB Angels Program, Little Rock, AR.)

recent study, patients with placenta accreta spectrum were managed either with usual care or with the online-to-offline model, where patients could reach providers instantly with WeChat. Based on interactions with the patients, physicians could initiate emergency plans for patients before patients even arrived to the hospital. This allowed for a reduction in time to emergent cesarean delivery from 50.7 minutes to 38.5 minutes.[40] A team in Colombia used telemedicine to train other physicians on conservative surgery as an option in management in cases of placenta accreta spectrum. Teleconsultation also was available intraoperatively. A center that did not previously perform conservative surgical management successfully performed 14 cases of conservative management, which allowed for safe uterine conservation.[41] Telemedicine can be used to manage care for placenta accreta spectrum and to allow for the utilization of alternative management.

mHealth also can be used to assist in caring for patients with diagnoses that are difficult to manage, such as human immunodeficiency virus (HIV). Coleman and colleagues[42] sent text messages 2 times weekly regarding pregnancy with support to 235 HIV-infected women. They compared outcomes with a control group of 586 patients who did not receive test messages. Women in the intervention group (text messaging) attended more antenatal visits, had increased chance of vaginal delivery, had decreased chance of a low-birth-weight infant, and were more likely to have their infant tested for HIV. Two text messages a week had a significant impact on maternal and child health in this cohort.

Telemedicine also can allow for monitoring of a high-risk pregnancy while the woman is at home. Morrison and colleagues[43] studied singleton gestations after discharge from the hospital. They performed daily uterine activity monitoring at home and had daily nursing contact. They found the telemedicine group had later gestational age at delivery, higher mean birth weight, fewer total nursery days, and decreased admissions to the neonatal intensive care unit. Lanssens and colleagues[44] performed a systematic review looking at the effectiveness of telemonitoring programs in preterm labor and observed that transmitting uterine activity resulted in significant prolongation of pregnancies.

SUMMARY

Telemedicine extends the reach of a health care system to beyond a typical brick and mortar building. Telemedicine visits, teleconsultations, teleultrasounds, and mHhealth applications all have merits in improving the current health care system, especially for those who are underserved. More research needs to be done on patient outcomes with telemedicine management of high-risk conditions.

ACKNOWLEDGMENTS

The authors would like to thank Ms Sheila L. Thomas, MA (LS), MEd, librarian at the University of Arkansas for Medical Sciences, for her valuable assistance with the literature search. The authors would also like to thank Ms Donna Eastham, BA, CRS, for her assistance with article editing and preparation.

DISCLOSURE

The authors have no commercial or financial conflicts of interest.

REFERENCES

1. Perednia DA, Allen A. Telemedicine technology and clinical applications. JAMA 1995;273(6):483–8.
2. van den Heuvel JF, et al. eHealth as the next-generation perinatal care: an overview of the literature. J Med Internet Res 2018;20(6):e202.
3. Rabie NZ, et al. Teleultrasound: how accurate are we? J Ultrasound Med 2017; 36(11):2329–35.
4. Buysse H, et al. Cost-effectiveness of telemonitoring for high-risk pregnant women. Int J Med Inform 2008;77(7):470–6.
5. CDC. Pregnancy-related deaths. 2019. Available at: https://www.cdc.gov/reproductivehealth/maternalinfanthealth/pregnancy-relatedmortality.htm. Accessed June 1, 2019.
6. Petersen EE, et al. Vital signs: pregnancy-related deaths, United States, 2011-2015, and strategies for prevention, 13 states, 2013-2017. MMWR Morb Mortal Wkly Rep 2019;68(18):423–9.
7. Steegers EA, et al. Pre-eclampsia. Lancet 2010;376(9741):631–44.
8. Ganapathy R, Grewal A, Castleman JS. Remote monitoring of blood pressure to reduce the risk of preeclampsia related complications with an innovative use of mobile technology. Pregnancy Hypertens 2016;6(4):263–5.
9. Lanssens D, et al. A prenatal remote monitoring program in pregnancies complicated with gestational hypertensive disorders: what are the contributors to the cost savings? Telemed J E Health 2019;25(8):686–92.

10. Lanssens D, et al. The impact of a remote monitoring program on the prenatal follow-up of women with gestational hypertensive disorders. Eur J Obstet Gynecol Reprod Biol 2018;223:72–8.

11. Dunsmuir DT, et al. Development of mHealth applications for pre-eclampsia triage. IEEE J Biomed Health Inform 2014;18(6):1857–64.

12. Hoppe KK, et al. Telehealth with remote blood pressure monitoring for postpartum hypertension: a prospective single-cohort feasibility study. Pregnancy Hypertens 2019;15:171–6.

13. Rhoads SJ, et al. Exploring implementation of m-health monitoring in postpartum women with hypertension. Telemed J E Health 2017;23(10):833–41.

14. Peterson C, et al. Preventable health and cost burden of adverse birth outcomes associated with pregestational diabetes in the United States. Am J Obstet Gynecol 2015;212(1):74.e1–9.

15. DeSisto CL, Kim SY, Sharma AJ. Prevalence estimates of gestational diabetes mellitus in the United States, pregnancy risk assessment monitoring system (PRAMS), 2007-2010. Prev Chronic Dis 2014;11:E104.

16. Mackillop L, et al. Development of a real-time smartphone solution for the management of women with or at high risk of gestational diabetes. J Diabetes Sci Technol 2014;8(6):1105–14.

17. Harrison TN, et al. Acceptability of virtual prenatal visits for women with gestational diabetes. Womens Health Issues 2017;27(3):351–5.

18. Ferrara A, et al. Referral to telephonic nurse management improves outcomes in women with gestational diabetes. Am J Obstet Gynecol 2012;206(6):491.e1–5.

19. Rasekaba TM, et al. Using technology to support care in gestational diabetes mellitus: quantitative outcomes of an exploratory randomised control trial of adjunct telemedicine for gestational diabetes mellitus (TeleGDM). Diabetes Res Clin Pract 2018;142:276–85.

20. Yang P, et al. Medical nutrition treatment of women with gestational diabetes mellitus by a telemedicine system based on smartphones. J Obstet Gynaecol Res 2018;44(7):1228–34.

21. Lau Y, et al. Efficacy of internet-based self-monitoring interventions on maternal and neonatal outcomes in perinatal diabetic women: a systematic review and meta-analysis. J Med Internet Res 2016;18(8):e220.

22. Ming WK, et al. Telemedicine technologies for diabetes in pregnancy: a systematic review and meta-analysis. J Med Internet Res 2016;18(11):e290.

23. Van Ryswyk EM, et al. Postpartum SMS reminders to women who have experienced gestational diabetes to test for Type 2 diabetes: the DIAMIND randomized trial. Diabet Med 2015;32(10):1368–76.

24. Salomon LJ, et al. Practice guidelines for performance of the routine midtrimester fetal ultrasound scan. Ultrasound Obstet Gynecol 2011;37(1):116–26.

25. Fisk NM, et al. Fetal telemedicine: six month pilot of real-time ultrasound and video consultation between the Isle of Wight and London. Br J Obstet Gynaecol 1996;103(11):1092–5.

26. Chan FY, et al. Clinical value of real-time tertiary fetal ultrasound consultation by telemedicine: preliminary evaluation. Telemed J 2000;6(2):237–42.

27. Long MC, Angtuaco T, Lowery C. Ultrasound in telemedicine: its impact in high-risk obstetric health care delivery. Ultrasound Q 2014;30(3):167–72.

28. Mistry H, Gardiner HM. The cost-effectiveness of prenatal detection for congenital heart disease using telemedicine screening. J Telemed Telecare 2013;19(4):190–6.

29. Brown J, Holland B. Successful fetal tele-echo at a small regional hospital. Telemed J E Health 2017;23(6):485–92.
30. Lowery C, et al. ANGELS and University of Arkansas for Medical Sciences paradigm for distant obstetrical care delivery. Am J Obstet Gynecol 2007;196(6): 534.e1–9.
31. Britt DW, Norton JD, Lowery CL. Equity in the development of telemedicine sites in an Arkansas high-risk pregnancy programme. J Telemed Telecare 2006;12(5): 242–5.
32. Bronstein JM, et al. Use of specialty OB consults during high-risk pregnancies in a Medicaid-covered population: initial impact of the Arkansas ANGELS intervention. Med Care Res Rev 2012;69(6):699–720.
33. Magann EF, et al. Evolving trends in maternal fetal medicine referrals in a rural state using telemedicine. Arch Gynecol Obstet 2012;286(6):1383–92.
34. Ivey TL, et al. Antenatal management of at-risk pregnancies from a distance. Aust N Z J Obstet Gynaecol 2015;55(1):87–9.
35. Rhoads SJ, et al. High-risk obstetrical call center: a model for regions with limited access to care. J Matern Fetal Neonatal Med 2018;31(7):857–65.
36. Britt DW, et al. A two-period assessment of changes in specialist contact in a high-risk pregnancy telemedical program. Telemed J E Health 2006;12(1):35–41.
37. Britt DW, Bronstein J, Norton JD. Absorbing and transferring risk: assessing the impact of a statewide high-risk-pregnancy telemedical program on VLBW maternal transports. BMC Pregnancy Childbirth 2006;6:11.
38. Wyatt SN, et al. Maternal response to high-risk obstetric telemedicine consults when perinatal prognosis is poor. Aust N Z J Obstet Gynaecol 2013;53(5):494–7.
39. Rabie NZ, et al. Prenatal diagnosis and telemedicine consultation of fetal urologic disorders. J Telemed Telecare 2016;22(4):234–7.
40. Sun W, et al. Comparison of maternal and neonatal outcomes for patients with placenta accreta spectrum between online-to-offline management model with standard care model. Eur J Obstet Gynecol Reprod Biol 2018;222:161–5.
41. Nieto-Calvache AJ, et al. Resective-reconstructive treatment of abnormally invasive placenta: Inter Institutional Collaboration by telemedicine (eHealth). J Matern Fetal Neonatal Med 2019;1–9. https://doi.org/10.1080/14767058.2019.1615877.
42. Coleman J, et al. Effectiveness of an SMS-based maternal mHealth intervention to improve clinical outcomes of HIV-positive pregnant women. AIDS Care 2017; 29(7):890–7.
43. Morrison J, et al. Telemedicine: cost-effective management of high-risk pregnancy. Manag Care 2001;10(11):42–6, 48-9.
44. Lanssens D, et al. Effectiveness of telemonitoring in obstetrics: scoping review. J Med Internet Res 2017;19(9):e327.

Clinical Applications of Telemedicine in Gynecology and Women's Health

Siwon Lee, MD, PhD, Wilbur C. Hitt, MD, FACOG FACOEM*

KEYWORDS

• Telemedicine • Telehealth • Gynecology • Well-woman visits

KEY POINTS

- Telemedicine is the practice of medicine using electronic information and telecommunication technologies from a distance.
- The use of telemedicine in gynecology is beneficial in screening, prevention, family planning, mental health, prescriptions, and procedures.
- Telemedicine will help patients and physicians in gynecology by increasing efficacy, extending the scope of practice, and improving outcomes.
- The future of telemedicine in gynecology is promising in terms of women's health care and gynecology surgery.

INTRODUCTION

Telemedicine and telehealth (TM/TH) are beneficial for patients living in remote and rural areas with limited medical resources. It is also practical for patients with rare or complex medical problems for which only subspecialists can recognize and treat. Local practitioners can get guidance and advice from a distant expert. The definition of telehealth is different from telemedicine because it contains a broader spectrum of distant health care services that involves remote "nonclinical" services.[1,2] For example, training health care providers, administrative meetings, medical education to providers and patients, in addition to clinical services, are examples of telehealth, whereas telemedicine only involves remote clinical services. The American Telemedicine Association and the World Health Organization (WHO) use the 2 terms interchangeably, focusing on the "remote" delivery of health care services as a critical factor.[1,2]

The history of telemedicine dates back to the 1950s. Telemedicine was first mentioned in a scientific article in 1974.[3,4] Telemedicine encompasses 3 methods of conveying information from a distant site: "store-and-forward," "real-time

Department of Obstetrics and Gynecology, Mount Sinai Medical Center, 4302 Alton Road, Suite 920, Miami Beach, FL 33140, USA
* Corresponding author.
E-mail address: Wchitt99@gmail.com

Obstet Gynecol Clin N Am 47 (2020) 259–270
https://doi.org/10.1016/j.ogc.2020.02.002
0889-8545/20/© 2020 Elsevier Inc. All rights reserved.

telemedicine," and "remote patient monitoring."[5] Store-and-forward involves acquiring medical information that is stored locally and subsequently sent to a specialist for interpretation later at a more convenient time. Real-time telemedicine provides real-time interactions between patients and physicians. Real-time interaction includes videoconferences, telephone, and online communications. In addition, the activities of history taking and physical examination can be done in an equivalent manner to the traditional on-site patient/physician interaction. With this method, the presence of both parties is required. With real-time interaction between the patient and physician, diagnosis and treatment can be offered to patients by virtual visits. Virtual visits permit patients with limited medical resources to access the care they need. Remote patient monitoring can be used for patients with chronic diseases, such as hypertension or diabetes. Examples of this type of monitoring include vital signs or blood glucose levels, which are transmitted to a provider electronically. This method can provide greater patient satisfaction as well as better health outcomes and is cost-effective.

Statistical data from the 2010 US County Census File for adult women (aged 15 years or older) and reproductive-aged women (15–44 years old) revealed that in the United States, there are 2.65 obstetrics and gynecology (OB-GYN) doctors for every 10,000 women and 5.39 OB-GYN doctors per 10,000 reproductive-aged women.[6] It is noteworthy that approximately 49% of all the US counties (3143) did not have a single OB-GYN doctor, and 8.2% of all US women lived in those predominantly rural counties.[7] Therefore, access to an OB-GYN specialist is challenging for the US population, especially in rural areas.

TM/TH can potentially improve access to general and specialty health services by reducing temporal and geographic barriers. With up-to-date technology, providers and patients will be able to communicate much more efficiently. Providers will have easier access to patient information, be able to conveniently update medical records, keep track of their patients, and write prescriptions. TM/TH will allow patients to check test results, request refills of prescriptions, review their medical record, view education materials, and even check in for appointments with mobile devices. The goal of TM/TH is to provide similar quality of care as the traditional physician/patient interaction but in a more economic and convenient manner. Patients do not have to miss work or travel great distances to have a physician/patient interaction. Remote patient monitoring should be able to detect problems earlier and result in fewer hospitalizations. All of these factors can result in a lower medical cost for both health care systems and patients.[1]

Unfortunately, some barriers and issues have kept TM/TH from expanding. TM/TH may disrupt the continuity of care because the patient might not be able to see the same health care provider every time. Sometimes diagnosis at a long distance will be difficult because some tests require additional equipment. Misdiagnosis because of distance or lack of information can lead to malpractice and legal problems. Finally, reimbursement for services can be an issue because there is no consensus about reimbursement between states and insurance companies, and this may be the biggest problem preventing TM/TH expansion.[1]

In gynecology, TM/TH can be used in many ways, including well-woman visits, preconception counseling (PCC), preventive care, infertility, psychiatry, family planning, teleradiology, and telesurgery.[5,8–11]

The purpose of this review is to summarize previously published literature on TM/TH applications to gynecology and women's health. The authors analyze the advantages and disadvantages of TM/TH in gynecology and suggest future applications to serve as a comprehensive source for new ideas.

WELL WOMAN'S VISIT AND PREVENTIVE CARE

Important features of a well-woman visit are a discussion of reproductive plans, care for women across her lifespan, and regular care for the perimenopausal and postmenopausal woman.

The well-woman visit consists of a screening for underlying medical conditions, maintenance of healthy life with preventive care, management of women at reproductive age with PCC, and referral to another specialist as needed. Indications for referral would include medical problems that require monitoring, history of pregnancy-related complications, and infertility. PCC is an excellent opportunity to counsel the patient on how to maintain a healthy lifestyle, improve her overall well-being, and provide preventive services.[8]

A head-to-toe physical examination was traditionally required during the well-woman visit. There are several instances whereby telemedicine can be a beneficial adjunct to the traditional physical examination. For example, the patient's history and review of system (ROS), follow-up of blood work, and additional screening tests are ideal for telemedicine.[8] A comprehensive history and ROS, including the gynecologic history, will give additional information to determine if the patient needs certain parts of the physical examination, such as a breast or pelvic examination. According to a recent American College of Obstetricians and Gynecologists (ACOG) committee opinion and a practice bulletin, pelvic and breast examinations are recommended only when indicated by medical history or symptoms.[12,13] A pelvic examination should be performed only after a thorough review of the patient's condition followed by a detailed discussion about risks and benefits of the examination between the health care provider and the patient.[12] There have been different opinions among the major groups that determine guideline recommendations for breast cancer screening.[14] ACOG's recommendations emphasize a shared decision making in choosing between the range of options recommended within different guidelines.[13]

The 2018 ACOG committee opinion on the annual well-woman examination recommended that the annual examination should include the woman's vital signs, body mass index (BMI), and assessment/management of the patient's health by screening, counseling, and immunizations based on the woman's age and risk factors.[8] OB-GYN doctors should be playing a critical role in engaging patients in shared decision making, encouraging healthy lifestyles, and counseling about effective preventive health practices.[8] Obtaining a family history is crucial in evaluating a patient's risk profile by identifying women at an increased risk for familial cancer. This early identification is important for optimal genetic testing and counseling; not uncommonly, there are some situations when it may not be possible to complete all of the recommended services in 1 visit or with 1 health care provider. TM/TH with team-based care, including the OB-GYN physicians, physician assistant (PA), nurse practitioner (NP), and other health care providers may facilitate meeting the needs of medical care for these women.

PRECONCEPTION COUNSELING

An important component of the well-woman visit for a reproductive-aged woman is a discussion about her life plan on reproduction. The patient can undergo screening and tests depending on her history, symptoms, and risk factors. This time is the ideal time when PCC, infertility assessment, health care related to sexually transmitted diseases, and a discussion on the full range of contraceptive options that are available can take place. The goal of PCC is not just to help a patient achieve pregnancy but to establish a favorable pregnancy outcome with a healthy mother and a baby.

PCC is an extension of a well-woman visit. A detailed discussion on lifestyle habits, body weight and nutrition, screening tests for antibody status that require vaccination as well as screening for a medical condition should be done in addition to routine gynecology testing. When something is detected or if the patient has known chronic medical conditions, these need to be addressed, controlled, and monitored. Reproductive history, including recurrent pregnancy loss (RPL), previous stillbirth, history of delivery of an infant with congenital anomalies, history of preterm labor, gestational diabetes, or preeclampsia, is meaningful information. Genetic counseling and screening can be offered to patients with increased risks of genetic disease.

Initial PCC using TM/TH can be either done with a general OB-GYN doctor, primary care physician (PCP), NP, or PA; then, if something abnormal is detected, the patient can be referred for specialist consultation using the TM/TH system. Ideal candidates for these consultations are women with known medical problems, for example, seizure disorders, blood clotting disorders, thyroid disease, chronic hypertension, diabetes, history of pregestational diabetes, poor obstetric history, and RPL. Assessment of body habitus can be done by calculating the BMI. Depending on BMI, the patient can be referred for counseling by a nutritionist and/or referral for bariatric treatment if appropriate.

TM/TH can be used not only for specialist consultation but also for general PCC. Lifestyle modifications, like smoking, alcohol, and recreational drug cessation, are a critical component of PCC and can be done using TM/TH.[15,16]

FAMILY PLANNING

Family planning is another essential component of the well-woman visit. When a woman reaches an age when contraception is important, it is crucial to counsel, educate, and provide the ideal form of contraception to each woman to maintain her optimal reproductive health. Nonetheless, getting an oral contraceptive (OCP) prescription has been the one of the greatest barriers to this population because of the difficulty in accessing physicians. According to a study in 2016, about 29% of women had difficulties in obtaining OCP prescriptions or refills.[9] The most common reasons were difficulty meeting a doctor, having no PCP or gynecologist, busy work schedule, and high medical costs.[9] Efforts to expand OCP prescription availability could be achieved by allowing a pharmacist to prescribe an OCP or making OCPs nonprescription drugs. Making OCPs nonprescription is realistically not possible because of the risks that could be caused by uncontrolled use of hormonal agents.[5,17] A newer effort to expand accessibility to OCPs is by using TM/TH to screen for medical conditions and provide a prescription. TM/TH has allowed a safe and effective way to provide education and prescription for contraception at an affordable cost with easier accessibility. Concerns have been voiced about the safety of using TM/TH to identify contraindications to the use of OCPs. Therefore, it is important to gather sufficient information using TM/TH to ensure that OCPS are safely prescribed.

INFERTILITY WORKUP

Team work is important for a comprehensive infertility workup. Reproductive endocrinology and infertility (REI) specialists, and PA, NP, embryologist, endocrine laboratory technician, nutritionist, psychiatrist, or psychologist are all part of the team that assists the women dealing with the physical and emotional aspects of infertility. Infertility treatment can involve multiple office visits, especially when patients are undergoing assisted reproductive technology. Currently, infertility management is generally not covered by most insurance carriers, which imposes a heavy burden in terms of time and money on the infertile couple. TM/TH can be helpful by reducing on-site visits when the physical encounter with the health care provider is not necessary.

Infertility management not only involves the general health management of the infertile woman but also may involve a genetic evaluation, mental illness counseling, detailed discussion about treatment options, laboratory tests, hysterosalpingography (HSG), ultrasound (US), and prescriptions for medications and injections before egg retrieval or embryo transfer procedures. One of the essential steps in the management of the infertility patient is the initial encounter between the physician and the patient. Usually, more than 30 minutes on average is necessary for a comprehensive history and ROS to understand the extent of what is involved in the couple's infertility.

Depression and anxiety are commonly present in many infertility patients. It has been reported that up to 40% of women with infertility have depression/anxiety, compared with a baseline rate of only 3% in the general population.[18] Although it is difficult to quantitate, stress appears to be a cause of infertility in some infertile women, and stress reduction has been shown to lead to an increased risk for a successful pregnancy.[10,19] Some previous studies have demonstrated that lifestyle modification programs and online psychoeducational support improved outcomes in patients with infertility by providing information and emotional support.[20–22]

In general, the initial infertility workup can be done by an OB-GYN generalist or another women's health care provider, but once an abnormal finding is identified, referral to an REI specialist is strongly recommended. Immediate referral to an REI specialist using TM/TH can reduce the overall medical cost, emotional stress, and time to conception.[23] At the initial evaluation, practitioners should make every effort not to order unnecessary tests. Usually, a full evaluation of a female patient begins from the onset of the menstrual period and needs a full menstrual cycle to complete. Once all female and male evaluations are completed, TM/TH consultation with REI specialist can be done to discuss the test results and the overall chance of achieving a healthy pregnancy and to set a realistic goal.

Currently, only psychoeducational support and teleradiology are actively used clinically in the TM/TH treatment of infertility. However, in the near future, using video conferencing with an REI specialist, medication prescription, and simple procedures that can be done under the guidance of a specialist will become possible. Video conferencing will result in fewer clinic visits and a reduction in the financial burden carried by infertility patients.

TELERADIOLOGY: ULTRASOUND

US is by far the safest, least invasive, and cost-effective imaging modality in gynecology. Conventional transvaginal 2-dimensional (2D) US is used to evaluate pelvic anatomy for suspected abnormalities in the uterus, fallopian tubes, and ovaries. Uterine leiomyoma, endometrial polyps, and ovarian or fallopian tube pathologic conditions can be detected with US. Recent advances in 3-dimensional and real-time 4-dimensional (3D/4D) US have added value to the evaluation of uterine anomalies or endometrial lesions. Telesonography has been used with obstetric US since 1997. Recent technology has made the assessment of the fetal heart remotely with real-time fetal echocardiogram using 4D spatiotemporal image correlation possible.[6] In gynecology, telesonography has had limited use. Although it may be early to incorporate TM/TH into routine clinical gynecologic practice, there has been a recent move toward using self-operated endovaginal telemonitoring and 3D/4D US for the assessment of the uterus in place of the traditional HSG in infertility patients. These studies have shown that using TM/TH technique was as accurate as the conventional in-person method, although more evidence-based studies need to be conducted to be applied in clinical practice.[24–26] Advantages of adding 3D/4D to 2D US are the ability to reconstruct an original image into any plane of choice, including the coronal plane, which is difficult with conventional 2D US. Other advantages of 3D/4D are no radiation exposure, easy accessibility, low cost, and the ability to operate from a long distance by another operator. these advantages are what makes the TM/TH system possible. TM/TH is an attractive option for assisting gynecologists in making diagnoses and making it easier for second opinions from specialists.

CERVICAL CANCER SCREENING AND COLPOSCOPY

Cervical cancer was the leading cause of cancer death for women in the Unites States. However, in the past 40 years, the number of cases and the number of deaths from cervical cancer have decreased significantly. This decline is the result of many women getting regular pap tests and human papillomavirus (HPV) testing, which can find a cervical precancerous lesion before it turns into cancer.[27,28] However, in developing countries with low medical resources, cervical cancer is still a major health challenge, with a high incidence and a high number of cancer-related deaths.[29–31] The problems in the developing countries are due to a lack in cervical cancer screening and follow up, problems with interpretation of the results of screening, and a lack of preventative education.

Following screening for cervical cancer with pap smears and/or HPV testing, colposcopy with or without biopsy may be indicated in some patients. Colposcopy is a simple method to diagnose cervical pathologic condition with a low-power binocular microscope and a high-intensity light source that can magnify the cervix. The most common indications for colposcopy are positive pap smears, positive HPV testing, and/or persistent unsatisfactory results from cytology. Acetowhite changes after acetic acid or changes in color to yellow or pale after Lugol solution are generally indications for biopsy of those sites. One of the problems with colposcopy is that significant pathologic changes can often be misinterpreted because of low specificity and high interobserver and intraobserver variability, which can only be achieved by proper training and good quality control.[32–34] Currently, in the United States, colposcopy training is only done during residency, and the Council on Resident Education in Obstetrics and Gynecology does not monitor how many cases of colposcopies are done to ensure proficiency during training. Compared with the United Kingdom, in the United States, there is no written certification examination or no standard curriculum for training colposcopy during residencies. This set of challenges results in a shortage of gynecologists properly trained in colposcopy. Because of a shortage of well-trained colposcopists, patients in areas with no specialists may have to travel great distances when they need a colposcopic evaluation. As a solution, the American Society for Colposcopy and Cervical Pathology published colposcopy standards recommendations in 2017 to influence the practice and to try and warrant quality assurance of colposcopy.[35,36] Another way to solve this problem is to use traditional binocular colposcopy combined with digital colposcopy using the TM/TH system. Colposcopy can be connected to a camera, and a still image or video images can be obtained and sent to the specialist for review.[5,37] The expert will review the images and give an opinion on the diagnosis and management as needed.[37] Nowadays, real-time assessment is even possible for the expert to review using video-conferencing technology, which enables the patient and physician to interact before, during, and after the procedure just as is done in an office setting.[38] The specialist will help guide the local practitioner to take the biopsies in the appropriate areas of concern. In previous studies, in-person examinations, real-time telecolposcopy, and store-and-forward of digital images were compared and showed a similar rate in the detection of cervical cancer. However, biopsy rates were higher in the store-and-forward group compared with on-site colposcopy.[39–41] TM/TH for colposcopy has the potential for improving the quality and reliability of the colposcopy, which would result in better counseling and teleconsulting with a gynecology oncologist when necessary. TM/TH will help reduce medical cost, improve quality control, and possibly decrease the level of interobserver variability.[5,32,42,43] Future large randomized trials will be needed to validate the validity of TM/TH for colposcopy. Overall, TM/TH can help improve capacity for colposcopy in areas without specialists and will be beneficial for inexperienced colposcopists who would benefit from the expertise of a specialist at a distance. TM/TH will make it possible for a more standardized practice of colposcopy using optimization of the document of colposcopic findings and assessment of competence of trainees.

MEDICAL ABORTION

Another essential aspect of family planning is the termination of pregnancy (TOP). According to WHO, the first-trimester TOP can be achieved on an outpatient basis by midlevel providers and by having the patient self-administer the medication and self-assess the abortion completeness at home.[44,45] There are limited data on the safety of medical abortion using TM/TH, but that data showed reassuring safety outcomes.[46,47] ACOG defines a medical abortion as the TOP before 10 weeks of gestation using mifepristone and misoprostol.[48] The efficacy of this regimen is approximately 92% in women with a gestation up to 49 days.[48] The first medical abortion using telemedicine occurred in 2008 at the Planned Parenthood of the Heartland facility in Iowa.[49] Using telemedicine as a means of TOP has increased the proportion of medical abortions undertaken before 12 weeks of gestation. TOP before 12 weeks is more likely to result in a complete abortion.[48,50] Studies have reported that medical abortions via telemedicine are as likely to be successful and to have a similar risk for adverse events as procedures done on site.[46,49]

MENTAL ILLNESSES IN GYNECOLOGY

Mental illness in gynecology can benefit from the use of TM/TH.[51] The prevalence of depression/anxiety is common in infertile women. Infertile women have comparable levels of anxiety and depression to those with heart disease, human immunodeficiency virus, or metastatic cancer.[9,10,52,53] Interventions that have included emotional support have been well researched and have shown favorable outcomes in this population. Psychological interventions may be offered in many forms, including individual counseling and therapy. Programs for infertile women that have provided counseling, personal attention, and support have shown a reduction in depression/anxiety and an increase in the pregnancy rate.[54,55] Recently, psychological interventions offered online have become popular. Studies comparing patients who received psychoeducational support through the Internet with patients who received no intervention showed that the intervention group had lower levels of depressive/anxiety symptoms and improved pregnancy rates after the intervention. This finding suggests that TM/TH maybe helpful in treating for mental illness in gynecology.[20–22,56]

PREOPERATIVE COUNSELING, POSTOPERATIVE CARE, AND TELESURGERY

TM/TH is currently used for preoperative and postoperative consultations, education on surgical procedures to patients, and teleconferencing locations with limited medical resources,[11] which has enabled patients to be able to make decisions on site rather than having to be transferred to larger facilities for education and consultations.[6] Routine postoperative care, using telemedicine, has been reported to be safe and effective.[11] TM/TH has allowed patients to be seen by specialists in distant sites without traveling to those sites, saving significant time and expense and resulting in increased patient satisfaction and reducing overall total medical cost.[11,57,58] Telemedicine, using videoconferencing, could also help physicians to assess minor complications and reduce unnecessary hospital visits.

Telesurgery is broadly defined as performing surgery from a distance[3] and is accomplished by supervising the surgery from a distance using real-time video-conference or performing the surgery using a robot. The first method can be used in remote or underserved areas where a specialist is not available to perform the procedure. In addition, it can be used in patients with a rare disease that requires specialist consultation. Multiple surgeons from different parts of the world can collaborate by a network to provide the best possible treatment for the individual patient, allowing not only the best care for the patient but also the exchange of ideas between physicians from anywhere in the world.[3,59] The second method involves robotic and telesurgical technology with minimally invasive gynecologic surgery. This method also enables the exchange of surgical techniques between the physicians and allows standardization of surgical training and better patient outcomes.[3] In gynecology, robotic-assisted surgery can be used in benign gynecology, gynecology oncology, reproductive endocrinology, and urogynecology. In a study comparing laparotomy with laparoscopy and robotic-assisted laparoscopy, the outcomes of wound complications (infectious and lung-related morbidity), postoperative ileus, and hematoma formation were compared between groups. There were more complications reported in the laparotomy group compared with the laparoscopy and robotic-assisted laparoscopy groups. No differences were noted between robotic-assisted and simple laparoscopic procedures, which could enable people in rural areas to have these surgeries using TM/TH.[60–62]

SUMMARY

With the rapid evolution of the Internet and information technology, TM/TH has evolved as a technology that is becoming more and more a part of the everyday practice of medicine in delivering high-quality health care.[11,63] Goals of TM/TH are not only improving the quality of medical care but also increasing convenience, increasing efficacy, and decreasing cost. TM/TH can be used as a cost-effective method of using medical resources and can lead to quick and reliable decisions. TM/TH is no longer a future medicine. Incorporating modern medicine into traditional in-person medicine is unavoidable. Now is the time for the health care providers to make changes in the mode of managing their patients. Telemedicine is one of the most rapidly growing areas in modern medicine, and many physicians see it as a method to increase efficiency, extend the scope of their practice, and improve outcomes. An important benefit of TM/TH is building a virtual community of physicians, thus facilitating discussion of their experiences, ideas, and cases in real time.

In gynecology, there is no doubt that TM/TH will play a crucial role in well-woman care. Although TM/TH looks very promising, some barriers require attention. For example, lack of in-person human interactions, misdiagnosis and malpractice insurance issues and legal issues, reimbursement and billing, problems with current state-specific medical licensing, and security of patient information are very important issues to be addressed and worked on before expansion of TM/TH. Although high-quality, large studies are still necessary to validate its efficacy and usefulness,

TM/TH has validated its value and advantages, especially in areas with limited medical resources.

DISCLOSURE

The authors have nothing to disclose.

REFERENCES

1. American Telemedicine Association. About telemedicine: the ultimate frontier for superior healthcare delivery. Available at: http://www.americantelemed.org/about-telemedicine. Accessed November 15, 2017.
2. World Health Organization. Telemedicine: opportunities and developments in member states. 2010. Available at: http://www.who.int/goe/publications/goe_telemedicine_2010.pdf. Accessed November 15, 2017.
3. Senapati S, Advincula A. Telemedicine and robotics: paving the way to the globalization of surgery. Int J Gynaecol Obstet 2005;91(3):210–6.
4. Zundel KM. Telemedicine: history, applications, and impact on librarianship. Bull Med Libr Assoc 1996;84(1):71.
5. Greiner AL. Telemedicine applications in obstetrics and gynecology. Clin Obstet Gynecol 2017;60(4):853–66.
6. Bullard TB, Rosenberg MS, Ladde J, et al. Digital images taken with a mobile phone can assist in the triage of neurosurgical patients to a level 1 trauma centre. J Telemed Telecare 2013;19(2):80–3.
7. Rayburn WF, Klagholz JC, Murray-Krezan C, et al. Distribution of American Congress of Obstetricians and Gynecologists fellows and junior fellows in practice in the United States. Obstet Gynecol 2012;119(5):1017–22.
8. Well-Woman visit. ACOG Committee opinion No. 755. American College of Obstetricians and Gynecologists. Obstet Gynecol 2018;132(4):e181–6.
9. Grindlay K, Grossman D. Prescription birth control access among US women at risk of unintended pregnancy. J Womens Health 2016;25(3):249–54.
10. Domar AD, Clapp D, Slawsby EA, et al. Impact of group psychological interventions on pregnancy rates in infertile women. Fertil Steril 2000;73(4):805–11.
11. Asiri A, AlBishi S, AlMadani W, et al. The use of telemedicine in surgical care: a systematic review. Acta Inform Med 2018;26(3):201.
12. The utility of and indications for routine pelvic examination. ACOG Committee Opinion No. 754. American College of Obstetricians and Gynecologists. Obstet Gynecol 2018;132:e174–80.
13. Breast cancer risk assessment and screening in average-risk women. Practice Bulletin No. 179. American College of Obstetricians and Gynecologists. Obstet Gynecol 2017;131:e1–16.
14. Center for Disease Control. Breast cancer screening guidelines for women. U.S. Preventive Services Task Force. 2016. American Cancer. Society. 2015. American College. Available at: https://www.cdc.gov/cancer/breast/pdf/BreastCancerScreeningGuidelines.pdf. Accessed November 15, 2017.
15. Gunatilake RP, Perlow JH. Obesity and pregnancy: clinical management of the obese gravida. Am J Obstet Gynecol 2011;204(2):106–19.
16. Vergel R, Sanchez L, Heredero B, et al. Primary prevention of neural tube defects with folic acid supplementation: Cuban experience. Prenat Diagn 1990;10(3):149–52.
17. Gomez AM. Availability of pharmacist-prescribed contraception in California, 2017. JAMA 2017;318(22):2253–4.

18. Chen T-H, Chang S-P, Tsai C-F, et al. Prevalence of depressive and anxiety disorders in an assisted reproductive technique clinic. Hum Reprod 2004;19(10): 2313–8.
19. van Dijk MR, Koster MP, Willemsen SP, et al. Healthy preconception nutrition and lifestyle using personalized mobile health coaching is associated with enhanced pregnancy chance. Reprod Biomed Online 2017;35(4):453–60.
20. Sexton MB, Byrd MR, O'Donohue WT, et al. Web-based treatment for infertility-related psychological distress. Arch Womens Ment Health 2010;13(4):347–58.
21. Cousineau TM, Green TC, Corsini E, et al. Online psychoeducational support for infertile women: a randomized controlled trial. Hum Reprod 2007;23(3):554–66.
22. Hämmerli K, Znoj H, Berger T. Internet-based support for infertile patients: a randomized controlled study. J Behav Med 2010;33(2):135–46.
23. VanderLaan B, Karande V, Krohm C, et al. Cost considerations with infertility therapy: outcome and cost comparison between health maintenance organization and preferred provider organization care based on physician and facility cost. Hum Reprod 1998;13(5):1200–5.
24. Saravelos SH, Jayaprakasan K, Ojha K, et al. Assessment of the uterus with three-dimensional ultrasound in women undergoing ART. Hum Reprod Update 2017;23(2):188–210.
25. Pereira I, von Horn K, Depenbusch M, et al. Self-operated endovaginal telemonitoring: a prospective, clinical validation study. Fertil Steril 2016;106(2):306–10.e1.
26. Wang Y, Qian L. Three- or four-dimensional hysterosalpingo contrast sonography for diagnosing tubal patency in infertile females: a systematic review with meta-analysis. Br J Radiol 2016;89(1063):20151013.
27. National Institutes of Health. Cervical cancer. NIH Consens Statement 1996; 14(1):1–38.
28. U.S. Cancer Statistics Working Group. U.S. Cancer statistics data visualizations tool, based on November 2018 submission data (1999-2016). Altlanta (GA): U.S. Department of Health and Human Services, Centers for Disease Control and Prevention and National Cancer Institute; 2019. Available at: www.cdc.gov/cancer/dataviz.
29. Stewart B, Wild CP. World cancer report 2014. Lyon (France): National Agency for Research on Cancer; 2014.
30. International Agency for Cancer Research. Globocan 2012—estimated cancer incidence, mortality and prevalence worldwide in 2012. Population fact sheets 2012. Available at: http://globocan.iarc.fr/Pages/fact_sheets_population.aspx#. Accessed October 28, 2015.
31. Linde DS, Andersen MS, Mwaiselage JD, et al. Text messages to increase attendance to follow-up cervical cancer screening appointments among HPV-positive Tanzanian women (Connected2Care): study protocol for a randomised controlled trial. Trials 2017;18(1):555.
32. Schaedel D, Kuehn W. The role of new information and communication technologies in gynecological diagnosis of cervical cancer. J Turk Ger Gynecol Assoc 2006;7(4):280–1.
33. Hopman EH, Voorhorst FJ, Kenemans P, et al. Observer agreement on interpreting colposcopic images of CIN. Gynecol Oncol 1995;58(2):206–9.
34. Etherington I, Luesley D, Shafi M, et al. Observer variability among colposcopists from the West Midlands region. BJOG 1997;104(12):1380–4.
35. Wentzensen N, Massad LS, Mayeaux EJ Jr, et al. Evidence-based consensus recommendations for colposcopy practice for cervical cancer prevention in the United States. J Low Genit Tract Dis 2017;21(4):216–22.

36. Mayeaux JE, Novetsky AP, Chelmow D, et al. ASCCP colposcopy standards: colposcopy quality improvement recommendations for the United States. J Low Genit Tract Dis 2017;21(4):242–8.

37. Hitt WC, Low GM, Lynch CE, et al. Application of a telecolposcopy program in rural settings. Telemed J E Health 2016;22(10):816–20.

38. Louwers J, Kocken M, Ter Harmsel W, et al. Digital colposcopy: ready for use? An overview of literature. BJOG 2009;116(2):220–9.

39. Hitt WC, Low G, Bird TM, et al. Telemedical cervical cancer screening to bridge Medicaid service care gap for rural women. Telemed J E Health 2013;19(5): 403–8.

40. Etherington IJ. Telecolposcopy—a feasibility study in primary care. J Telemed Telecare 2002;8(2_suppl):22–4.

41. Ferris DG, Bishai DM, Litaker MS, et al. Telemedicine network telecolposcopy compared with computer-based telecolposcopy. J Low Genit Tract Dis 2004; 8(2):94–101.

42. Ricard-Gauthier D, Wisniak A, Catarino R, et al. Use of smartphones as adjuvant tools for cervical cancer screening in low-resource settings. J Low Genit Tract Dis 2015;19(4):295–300.

43. Spitzer M. The era of "digital colposcopy" will be here soon. J Low Genit Tract Dis 2015;19(4):273–4.

44. Endler M, Lavelanet A, Cleeve A, et al. Telemedicine for medical abortion: a systematic review. BJOG 2019;126(9):1094–102.

45. World Health Organization. Health worker roles in providing safe abortion care and post-abortion contraception. Geneva (Switzerland): World Health Organization; 2015.

46. Grossman D, Grindlay K. Safety of medical abortion provided through telemedicine compared with in person. Obstet Gynecol 2017;130(4):778–82.

47. Aiken AR, Digol I, Trussell J, et al. Self reported outcomes and adverse events after medical abortion through online telemedicine: population based study in the Republic of Ireland and Northern Ireland. BMJ 2017;357:j2011.

48. Medical management of first-trimester abortion. Practice Bulletin No 143. American College of Obstetricians and Gynecologists. Obstet Gynecol 2014;123: 676–92.

49. Grossman D, Grindlay K, Buchacker T, et al. Effectiveness and acceptability of medical abortion provided through telemedicine. Obstetrics Gynecol 2011; 118(2):296–303.

50. Grossman DA, Grindlay K, Buchacker T, et al. Changes in service delivery patterns after introduction of telemedicine provision of medical abortion in Iowa. Am J Public Health 2013;103(1):73–8.

51. Douglas MD, Xu J, Heggs A, et al. Assessing telemedicine utilization by using Medicaid claims data. Psychiatr Serv 2016;68(2):173–8.

52. Domar AD, Broome A, Zuttermeister PC, et al. The prevalence and predictability of depression in infertile women. Fertil Steril 1992;58(6):1158–63.

53. Domar AD, Zuttermeister P, Friedman R. The psychological impact of infertility: a comparison with patients with other medical conditions. J Psychosom Obstet Gynaecol 1993;14:45–52.

54. Domar AD, Rooney KL, Wiegand B, et al. Impact of a group mind/body intervention on pregnancy rates in IVF patients. Fertil Steril 2011;95(7):2269–73.

55. Terzioglu F. Investigation into effectiveness of counseling on assisted reproductive techniques in Turkey. J Psychosom Obstet Gynaecol 2001;22(3):133–41.

56. Clifton J, Parent J, Worrall G, et al. An internet-based mind/body intervention to mitigate distress in women experiencing infertility: a randomized pilot trial. Fertil Steril 2016;106(3):e62.

57. Costa MA, Yao CA, Gillenwater TJ, et al. Telemedicine in cleft care: reliability and predictability in regional and international practice settings. J Craniofac Surg 2015;26(4):1116–20.

58. Urquhart AC, Antoniotti NM, Berg RL. Telemedicine—an efficient and cost-effective approach in parathyroid surgery. Laryngoscope 2011;121(7):1422–5.

59. Rafiq A, Merrell RC. Telemedicine for access to quality care on medical practice and continuing medical education in a global arena. J Contin Educ Health Prof 2005;25(1):34–42.

60. Cho J, Shamshirsaz A, Nezhat C, et al. New technologies for reproductive medicine: laparoscopy, endoscopy, robotic surgery and gynecology. A review of the literature. Minerva Ginecologica 2010;62(2):137–67.

61. Stark M, Benhidjeb T, Gidaro S, et al. The future of telesurgery: a universal system with haptic sensation. J Turk Ger Gynecol Assoc 2012;13(1):74.

62. Haidegger T, Sándor J, Benyó Z. Surgery in space: the future of robotic telesurgery. Surg Endosc 2011;25(3):681–90.

63. World Health Organization, Region Office for Europe. From innovation to implementation eHealth in the WHO European Region. Available at: http://www.euro.who.int/_data/assets/pdf_file/0012/302331?From-Innovation-to-Implementation-eHealth-Report-EU.pdf. Accessed March 18, 2018.

Telemedicine and Gynecologic Cancer Care

David I. Shalowitz, MD, MSHP[a,b],*, Catherine J. Moore, BS[a]

KEYWORDS

- Gynecologic cancer • Telemedicine • Teleoncology • Cancer care delivery research
- Access to care

KEY POINTS

- Significant outcomes disparities exist for patients with gynecologic cancers based on place of residence.
- Telemedicine may decrease or eliminate geographic barriers to high-quality gynecologic cancer care.
- Telemedical applications exist for the prediagnosis, pretreatment, treatment, and post-treatment/survivorship phases of cancer care.
- Implementation of telemedical cancer care requires consideration of all stakeholders' needs.

INTRODUCTION

In 2020, approximately 113,520 new cases of gynecologic cancers will be diagnosed, and approximately 33,620 women will die from these diseases. The incidence and mortality are predicted to be highest for cancers of the ovary (21,750 cases and 13,940 deaths), uterine corpus (65,620 cases and 12,590 deaths), and uterine cervix (13,800 cases and 4,290 deaths) with the remainder attributed to malignancies of the vulva, vagina, and other genital sites.[1] From 2005 to 2015, the incidence of uterine corpus cancer increased from 25.0 to 27.7 cases per 100,000 women; the incidence of ovarian cancer increased from 10.7 to 12.0 cases per 100,000. Over the same time period, the incidence of cervical cancer remained stable, with an estimated 6.8 cases per 100,000 women in 2015. Although the death rate from ovarian cancer has decreased from 8.8 to 7.1 per 100,000 from 2005 to 2015, the combined death rate over the same interval from cancers of the uterine corpus and cervix has increased from 6.5 to 7.1 per 100,000.[2]

[a] Section on Gynecologic Oncology, Department of Obstetrics and Gynecology, Wake Forest School of Medicine, Winston-Salem, NC, USA; [b] Department of Implementation Sciences, Wake Forest University School of Medicine, Winston-Salem, NC, USA
* Corresponding author. Section on Gynecologic Oncology, 4th Floor Watlington Hall, Medical Center Boulevard, Winston-Salem, NC 27157.
E-mail address: dshalowi@wakehealth.edu

Obstet Gynecol Clin N Am 47 (2020) 271–285
https://doi.org/10.1016/j.ogc.2020.02.003
0889-8545/20/© 2020 Elsevier Inc. All rights reserved.

obgyn.theclinics.com

Disparities in survival outcomes after a diagnosis of gynecologic cancers have been clearly and consistently associated with race, rural residence, socioeconomic status, comorbidities, tumor biology, and preventative behaviors, for example, vaccination for the human papillomavirus to decrease the risk of cervical cancer.[3,4] Of these, telemedicine is best suited to help overcome geographic barriers to care experienced by women with gynecologic cancers.

GEOGRAPHIC DISPARITIES IN GYNECOLOGIC CANCER CARE

Rural populations have a higher incidence of cervical cancer,[5] are less likely to undergo ovarian cancer surgery by a gynecologic oncologist,[6] and may experience worsened survival with ovarian cancer.[7,8] Rural residence is also associated with a decreased likelihood of undergoing comprehensive surgical treatment for endometrial cancer and worsened survival associated with the disease.[9] Increasing distance from residence to a specialty care center may also be associated with decreased likelihood of receiving care consistent with national guidelines, for example, those published by the National Comprehensive Cancer Network, and subsequent worsened survival. This relationship seems to be particularly strong for patients with ovarian cancer[10]; data conflict for patients with endometrial and cervical cancers.[11–14]

It is challenging to interpret associations between distance traveled for care and clinical outcomes for 3 reasons. First, patients may bypass cancer care at the closest available center if a distant center is perceived to be superior, if there is no insurance coverage for the closest institution, or if they are unaware of the closest institution.[15] Second, most analyses of the relationship between distance traveled for cancer care and outcomes are abstracted from state registries that are limited by boundaries, and therefore cannot consider patients who cross state lines for treatment.[10] Third, there is evidence of an urban–rural paradox in patients with cervical cancer; although rural populations are likely to have worse outcomes overall, increased distance to care may be a greater barrier for urban populations than rural populations.[16] This phenomenon suggests that there may be a benefit to equalizing geographic disparities within both urban and rural populations. The decision processes used by patients to choose a hospital for their cancer treatment remain unclear and are an area of active investigation.[17]

In the United States, the standard of care for patients with gynecologic cancers includes consultation with a gynecologic oncologist.[18–21] Unfortunately, many women are at risk for geographic barriers to access to care based on distance to the nearest gynecologic oncologist.[22,23] There is emerging evidence that equalizing access to care may decrease, if not negate, some geographic disparities. For example, in 1 national sample, disparities in cervical cancer incidence between rural and urban populations was statistically explained by geographic access to health care providers.[24] An analysis of data from New York suggested that outcomes for rural patients with cervical and endometrial cancers improved with expansion of access to detection and treatment of early-stage disease, presumably by providers of primary and general gynecologic care. However, similar improvement was not seen in outcomes for rural patients with ovarian cancer, likely because early diagnosis is challenging and appropriate treatment generally requires referral for expert surgical and chemotherapeutic management.[14] Another study conducted within the Southwest Oncology Group found that urban–rural disparities in survival outcomes were equalized when patients were treated on a clinical trial.[25] Furthermore, no racial differences in survival outcomes existed among patients treated for cervical cancer within the US Military Health System, within which access to treatment is guaranteed regardless of geography.[26]

Telemedicine is essential to improve care delivery for women with gynecologic cancers at risk for geographic survival disparities. Although some commentators advocate for improving gynecologic cancer outcomes by consolidating care in high-volume referral centers,[27,28] this approach is likely to be challenging in the United States. Of patients with ovarian cancer. 25% to 35% are currently cared for in low-volume settings[29,30]; redistributing this population's care to referral centers may carry significant travel burdens for patients, and it is unclear that patients are willing to travel for treatment, even for improved survival outcomes.[17] Additionally, although oncologists may travel to rural sites,[31] this approach is inefficient and burdensome[32] and cannot cover the nearly 60% of the United States located more than 50 miles from the nearest gynecologic oncologist.[22] It is therefore critical to invest in telemedical infrastructure to allow patients with gynecologic cancers maximal access to the benefits of subspecialty care while minimizing the burdens of potentially unnecessary travel.

Although telemedicine is generally used to extend referral centers' catchment to rural areas, telemedicine may also be used to expand access for patients for whom any travel is prohibitive, including those with substantial comorbidities or requiring end-of-life care. Likewise, the findings of an urban–rural paradox suggest that access to cancer care could be improved by minimizing travel needed for urban patients. Even though these patients may reside substantially closer to referral institutions than their rural counterparts, socioeconomic factors may be a greater barrier to travel than distance.

RESOURCES REQUIRED FOR HIGH-QUALITY GYNECOLOGIC CANCER CARE

High-quality care for patients with gynecologic cancers requires coordination among providers from multiple specialties. Consultation with a gynecologic oncologist remains the cornerstone of gynecologic cancer care, based on improved outcomes related to uniquely specialized training in the surgical and medical treatment of these diseases.[33] Patients may also benefit from access to pathologists,[34] radiation oncologists,[35] diagnostic radiologists,[36] palliative care providers,[37] genetic counselors,[38] and patient navigators[39] with expertise in gynecologic cancers. Depending on individual patients' circumstances, these providers may need to coordinate any of a range of services, including:

- Review of radiologic or pathologic studies, or physical examination findings,
- Treatment planning in a multidisciplinary tumor board,
- Surgery by a high-volume surgeon with a minimally invasive approach if appropriate,
- Radiation therapy, including external beam and/or brachytherapy,
- Medical treatment, including chemotherapy, immunotherapy, and hormonal therapies,
- Counseling regarding the implications of germline and tumor genetic testing,
- Palliative and end-of-life care, and
- Clinical trial enrollment.

We previously described the continuum of care for gynecologic malignancies as including 4 distinct phases. The prediagnosis phase ends when a cancer diagnosis is made; the pretreatment phase begins after diagnosis and ends with initiation of treatment; the treatment phase begins with initiation of treatment and ends when treatment has been completed; the post-treatment/survivorship phase begins after completion of treatment and ends with resumption of treatment or death.[40] It is helpful to consider the elements of cancer care within each of these phases alongside applications of telemedicine to link patients with providers and services.

BEFORE DIAGNOSIS

Whenever possible, premalignant lesions and early-stage malignancies should be detected and managed through appropriate screening protocols and prompt evaluation of concerning symptoms. The application of telemedicine to routine gynecologic care, including cancer screening, is discussed detail in Siwon Lee and Wilbur C. Hitt's article, "Clinical Applications of Telemedicine in Gynecology and Women's Health," elsewhere in this issue.

The prediagnosis phase of care may include a telemedical consultation to establish a diagnosis or to determine whether subspecialty referral is needed. It may sometimes be unclear whether a specimen is diagnostic of a malignant or premalignant condition. Pathways for pathologic consultation are generally well-established, and samples can usually be sent to outside experts for review when required. Remote examination of frozen section specimens can be used when local intraoperative pathologic expertise is not available and has excellent diagnostic accuracy.[41] Likewise, remote review of radiologic images is very well-established as a means to expand access to radiologic care.[42]

A curbside consultation[43] platform may facilitate communication or review of patient data between general practitioners or nononcologic specialists and oncology specialists, without in-person or virtual patient contact. Communication between gynecologic cancer specialists and other providers, including general obstetrician-gynecologists, primary care providers, emergency medicine physicians, and medical or surgical oncologists, is critical to ensure that diagnoses are made in a timely fashion. Curbsides may also be used to determine whether a patient requires referral, whether surgical intervention is recommended, and whether surgery is best undertaken by a specialist (eg, a gynecologic oncologist) or by a general surgeon or gynecologist. Importantly, some patients should be referred to a gynecologic oncologist *before* a diagnosis has been made; for example, the American College of Obstetricians and Gynecologists recommends that patients with a suspicious pelvic mass should be evaluated by a gynecologic oncologist, even though a substantial proportion of these patients will not have malignant disease on final surgical pathology.[20]

The Association of American Medical Colleges has piloted an electronic platform to facilitate access to specialists' recommendations by primary care providers.[44] This infrastructure is likely to be easily applicable to virtual consultations across different subspecialties (eg, medical oncologist to gynecologic oncologist) or from a specialist to a subspecialist (eg, obstetrician-gynecologist to gynecologic oncologist). Once established, virtual networks linking specialists and general practitioners can disseminate guidelines regarding diagnosis, screening, and management of malignant and premalignant gynecologic diseases. The experience of the ECHO program administered by the University of New Mexico for select nononcologic care scenarios may be adaptable for this purpose.[45] Ongoing communication between specialists in gynecologic cancer care and other care providers, whether formally or informally related to a patient, or for educational purposes, promotes effective and efficient use of providers' time and potentially saves patients from unnecessary travel for in-person evaluation.

BEFORE TREATMENT

The majority of time spent in the pretreatment phase of care is occupied by treatment planning and preparation. Once a gynecologic cancer has been diagnosed, patients may benefit from a multidisciplinary treatment planning conference, or tumor board, including gynecologic oncologists, medical oncologists, radiation oncologists, radiologists, and pathologists. Telemedical infrastructure, including videoconferencing, can link physicians in outlying hospitals to specialists at a cancer referral center. Two promising pilot studies suggest that telemedical tumor boards for gynecologic cancers are feasible and associated with improvements in patient care.[46,47]

Depending on the treatment plan and available local personnel, an initial consultation may be in person with subsequent encounters performed virtually, or all interaction with a specialist may be virtual with subsequent treatment administered by a local provider.[48] Although patients with cancer may prefer to undergo a physical examination by the specialist oncologist,[49,50] a systematic review of 19 trials including 709 patients suggested that outcomes are not compromised by virtual visits and that physicians and patients are satisfied with remote interaction.[51] These findings are likely generalizable across outpatient and inpatient settings. Remote preoperative consultation was feasible and saved costs in a surgical oncology practice within the Veterans Health Administration system.[52] In a pediatric surgery population, preoperative examinations were noted to be especially helpful with an experienced on-site examiner during the virtual consultation.[53] It is unclear how these data may apply to the preoperative evaluation of patients with gynecologic malignancies. In many cases, imaging may guide the surgical approach, although physical examination by an expert surgeon may be indispensable for the evaluation of cervical pathology and for determining the need for gastrointestinal or urinary procedures as a part of cytoreduction. For patients with an increased perioperative risk, preoperative medical evaluation, clearance, and optimization may be done locally or remotely, depending on the preference and capability of the treating institution's anesthesiologists.[54]

There is concern that the association between delayed treatment after a diagnosis of gynecologic cancer and worsened survival may be related to barriers to accessing subspecialty care.[55] In theory, establishing clinical and educational communication networks between gynecologic cancer specialists and the diagnosing providers may facilitate more rapid evaluation and initiation of treatment, although this effect has not been studied.

TREATMENT

Treatment of gynecologic cancers may involve a combination of surgical, medical, and radiotherapeutic modalities. In addition, patients may benefit from supportive and palliative care services, and enrollment in clinical trials.

Surgery is the most difficult component of cancer care to provide remotely. The technical feasibility of surgery by a remote operator was established in 2002[56]; current areas of emphasis in telesurgery research include decreasing the duration and impact of communication latency between the remote operator and the surgical platform,[57,58] improved haptic feedback,[59] and improved portability of the point-of-care surgical platform.[60] Unfortunately, true telesurgery currently requires a robotic platform that is expensive, not easily transported, and consequently not easily adapted to the rural setting. The routine use of telesurgery for gynecologic cancers consequently remains experimental.

In some cases, a specialist might provide intraoperative guidance to a remote surgeon. When used as a training aid, telementoring can increase surgeons' comfort with new procedures and is associated with equivalent outcomes to in-person training.[61] The same infrastructure may be used episodically for intraoperative consultation; real-time availability of a remote surgical consultant might improve the rate at which surgeons without significant experience treating gynecologic cancers adequately treat these malignancies. It remains to be seen whether telementoring would thereby improve access to appropriate surgical care, decrease the need for adjuvant therapies, or improve survival outcomes. Currently, therefore, patients requiring radical, staging, or cytoreductive procedures for gynecologic cancers are best served by high-volume surgeons at institutions experienced in the management of these cases. Telemedical triage of cases may allow patients with some conditions to undergo surgery locally with subsequent referral to a specialist as needed.[62]

There is good support for the feasibility and effectiveness of monitoring postoperative patients remotely.[63] In one study, mental health scores improved after ovarian cancer surgery with the use of a web-based monitoring application; however, physical health scores decreased, possibly owing to patients' increased awareness of symptoms.[64] Mobile phone-based monitoring for postoperative patients after nongynecologic cancer surgery improved follow-up rates, as well as fewer readmissions and unscheduled visits to the clinic or emergency department.[65,66] Smartphone-based wound monitoring in general surgical populations can improve access to care for rural patients.[67,68] Treatment decisions made during video-based postoperative visits were highly concordant with decisions made in person and were associated with a high degree of patient satisfaction.[69,70]

The application of telemedicine to support the remote management of medical treatment for rural patients with cancer was pioneered in the United States by the University of Kansas,[71] and in Australia by the Townsville Cancer Center in Queensland.[72] These practices use remote consultation, prescription, and supervision of chemotherapy by an oncologist, with on-site drug administration by local nursing staff. Remote administration of chemotherapy was associated with similar safety and patient satisfaction to treatment at the referral center.[72,73] Although these populations do not include patients with gynecologic cancers, the same principles of remote supervision of chemotherapy apply. Likewise, the experience gained with cytotoxic chemotherapy should translate to remote supervision of targeted therapies (eg, poly adenosine diphosphate-ribose polymerase inhibitors), as well as hormonal, antiangiogenic, and immunologic therapies. Remote genetic counseling protocols are relatively well-developed and may be an important resource for patients without local access to a genetic counselor.[74]

Two systematic reviews suggest that electronic symptom monitoring may improve quality of life for patients with cancer[75,76]; a third review suggested that the strength of support for Internet-based interventions for chemotherapy-related symptoms was limited by studies' methodology.[77] Two studies involving patients with gynecologic cancers undergoing surgery[78] or chemotherapy[79] found benefit with remote symptom monitoring. Telemedical technology can provide access to palliative care and symptom management from patients' homes, and decrease emergency room visits and unplanned admissions, although there is concern that adequate care for some complex patients with cancer may be infeasible without an in-person visit.[80] Oncologists should be cautious when considering addition of routine telemedical encounters for symptom management, because these may paradoxically worsen patients' quality of life by drawing attention to symptoms.[81] When a visit to an emergency department is unavoidable, a telemedical consultation with a gynecologic cancer specialist may allow for local treatment without the need for a costly transfer.[82]

Radiation therapy for gynecologic cancers requires significant investment in equipment, infrastructure, and personnel. Consequently, institutions capable of administering radiation therapy likely have radiation oncology and medical physics staff on site. The greatest impact of telemedicine on radiation therapy has been the ability to expand access by triaging cases within a tiered system of care: patients determined to be low complexity may be treated at outlying centers, whereas patients who may benefit from higher complexity treatment plans (eg, involving brachytherapy or intensity-modulated therapy) are treated at a referral center.[83] Teleradiotherapy has also been successfully implemented for patient consultation and follow-up related to radiation treatments, building on the success of teleconsultation for medical oncology visits.[84] Furthermore, remote review and automated treatment planning for patients with cervical cancer may allow more patients to be treated in low-resource settings where the number of patients treated is limited by radiation therapy staff.[85]

The application of telemedicine to patient enrollment and participation in cancer-related clinical trials is poorly studied. Ideally, patients should have access to trials of novel therapeutics, regardless of where they reside. Practically, the expansion of clinical trials to rural or satellite sites would likely involve additional personnel, inclusion of telemedical methods study protocols, verification of clinical practices at outlying sites, and potentially budgeting for equipment to allow for telemedical consultation.[86] However, these barriers might be overcome and certainly deserve further study. The National Cancer Institute's Community Oncology Research Program may be a promising platform to study the implementation of telemedicine for enrollment of gynecologic patients with cancer in clinical trials.[40]

AFTER TREATMENT AND SURVIVORSHIP

After treatment has concluded, gynecologic cancer care generally involves surveillance for recurrent or progressive disease, and for those patients with active disease who are not candidates for treatment, continued symptom management and end-of-life care. Guidelines for surveillance of patients with a history of gynecologic cancer emphasize screening for symptoms and physical examination findings concerning for recurrent disease.[87] These elements of survivorship care may be performed by any provider able to detect abnormalities on general and pelvic examinations; the assistance of gynecologic cancer specialists may be enlisted for interpretation of tumor markers and imaging results. As in the prediagnosis and pretreatment phases, a gynecologic cancer specialist should be consulted either in person or virtually whenever there is concern for recurrent disease. The creation and maintenance of virtual networks between gynecologic cancer specialists and nononcologic care providers may facilitate referral when clinically indicated, and save patients the burdens of travel for routine visits.

Finally, telemedicine has great potential to increase access to hospice and end-of-life care for rural patients and other patients for whom in-person evaluation by hospice services is not available. The evidence base for these interventions is, however, not yet fully developed.[88,89] Importantly, the use of telemedicine for hospice and end-of-life care is likely to require clinicians to interact primarily with patients' caregivers, depending on the patient's ability to communicate.

STAKEHOLDER CONSIDERATIONS

The implementation of a telemedical program for gynecologic cancer care requires a careful stakeholder analysis. Acceptance of the program by 4 groups is essential: patients, gynecologic oncologists, referring physicians, and administrators of the health system(s) within which the program is located. Although some details will be specific to local needs, the following themes should be considered.

For patients, considerations involve the burdens of travel for care, benefits associated with specialist referrals, and quality of the patient–physician relationship. In the United States, burdens associated with travel are highly variable and depend on geography and population density. Barriers to travel may include distance, traffic, infrastructure (eg, highway vs local roads), topography, or weather (eg, mountain roads rendered impassable in winter). Additionally, some patients may have variable access to transportation, depend on public transportation, or have comorbidities that make travel challenging regardless of distance or mode of travel. Although the goal of implementing telemedicine for gynecologic cancer care is to allow patients access to improved outcomes from specialized care, a substantial proportion of patients may prefer not to engage with specialists for unclear reasons.[17] It is therefore critical to ensure sufficient buy-in from potential patients when planning to implement telemedical cancer care. Likewise, from patients' perspectives, there must be sufficient benefit to participate in an alternative model of care. Relevant benefits might include improved clinical outcomes, quality of life, or convenience. Communication between the health system providing telemedical cancer care and the physicians and patients using telemedicine will be critical to ensuring that there is sufficient perceived benefit to promote continued use. Finally, patients may be concerned about the quality of the provider–patient relationship if their care is managed remotely. Although the available data suggest that this concern may be overcome, the type of interaction patients prefer may vary by population and location, and should be considered carefully when developing telemedical procedures.

For gynecologic cancer specialists, including gynecologic oncologists, telemedicine offers the prospect of increasing case volume by expanding the catchment area served without requiring outreach travel by providers. Additionally, facilitated communication (eg, through a curbside consultation platform) with referring providers likely allows specialists to select for formal consultation only those patients who fit most with their desired scope of practice. For example, a gynecologic oncologist might be able to increase her ability to evaluate new patients with cancer by triaging patients with benign disease to general gynecologists before a referral is made. Cancer specialists need to be confident that the telemedical program does not overly impair the provider–patient relationship or prevent the delivery of high-quality care. Providers' usability of the telemedical interface should be prioritized to avoid the professional burnout strongly associated with use of electronic medical record systems.[90] Likewise, the reimbursement schema for participation in telemedical cancer care must be perceived as fair to ensure equal prioritization of patients managed remotely and in person.

Noncancer specialists referring into the telemedical program for gynecologic cancer care are likely vested in the program's ability to provide efficient responses to clinical questions not requiring immediate referral to a cancer specialist, expeditious evaluation of patients who are referred, and the availability of education on relevant diagnosis and management skills for their practice. Care providers with a longitudinal relationship with patients with cancer may appreciate the opportunity to manage patients under the guidance of a cancer specialist (eg, routine examinations during survivorship). These providers will also likely appreciate the ability to receive updates on a patient's cancer treatment, whether through an electronic medical record or otherwise. Reimbursement to these providers for participating in the telemedical program may also improve uptake and satisfaction with this model of care.

Finally, the successful implementation of a telemedical program for gynecologic cancer care requires substantial investment by health systems and payers. Cost-effectiveness analyses will assist in motivating these parties to invest in developing and maintaining telemedicine programs.[91] For insurers offering narrow network health plans, the use of telemedicine may satisfy state or federal network adequacy requirements for access to cancer care.[92] Both payers and health systems may be motivated by the prospect of increasing market share of patients with gynecologic cancers through virtual outreach and care structures, and with the marketing benefit that may accompany the availability of virtual outreach.

IMPLEMENTATION AND NEXT STEPS

Given the complex interplay of multiple stakeholders in providing gynecologic cancer care, health systems considering implementation of a telemedical program should consider carefully the goals that such a program is intended to achieve. Short-term and long-term goals for each health system may differ; these goals may determine which elements of the program are implemented first and which are added subsequently. For example, a health system might prioritize advertising the rapid availability of gynecologic oncologists for consultation by obstetrician-gynecologists and initiate a virtual curbside consultation platform as a first step. Virtual, formal consultation, and patient management services would be added to the program subsequently, once referral pathways and relationships with outlying providers were established.

It is absolutely critical to emphasize the perceived usefulness and ease of use of new telemedical systems. Specifically, individuals involved must feel that elements of the telemedical program both allow them to accomplish their goals more easily than alternatives (ie, providing or receiving cancer care), and are relatively uncomplicated to use.[93] This may require multiple rounds of pilot testing and substantial upfront investment in ensuring adequate interoperability with existing electronic medical record and imaging systems. Likewise, billing and reimbursement for participation in telemedical programs should be transparent to providers. Although regulations regarding the reimbursement of telemedicine are complex (and discussed in Janet L. McCauley and colleagues' article, "Reframing Telehealth: Regulation, Licensing, and Reimbursement in Connected Care," in this issue), at the very least, providers should not feel that they may be penalized for investing their time in adopting a new method of cancer care.

SUMMARY

Telemedicine holds the promise of substantially decreasing the impact of geographic disparities in the outcomes of gynecologic cancers by decreasing barriers to accessing specialty cancer care. Health systems should strongly consider prioritizing the integration of telemedicine into cancer care to ensure that women with gynecologic malignancies are able to benefit from high-quality care regardless of where they reside.

DISCLOSURE

The authors report no conflicts of interest.

REFERENCES

1. Siegel RL, Miller KD, Jemal A. Cancer statistics, 2019. CA Cancer J Clin 2019; 69(1):7–34.
2. American Cancer Society Cancer Statistics Center. Available at: https:// cancerstatisticscenter.cancer.org/#!/. Accessed May 10, 2017.

3. Collins Y, Holcomb K, Chapman-Davis E, et al. Gynecologic cancer disparities: a report from the Health Disparities Taskforce of the Society of Gynecologic Oncology. Gynecol Oncol 2014;133(2):353–61.

4. Temkin SM, Rimel BJ, Bruegl AS, et al. A contemporary framework of health equity applied to gynecologic cancer care: a Society of Gynecologic Oncology evidenced-based review. Gynecol Oncol 2018;149(1):70–7.

5. Zahnd WE, James AS, Jenkins WD, et al. Rural–urban differences in cancer incidence and trends in the United States. Cancer Epidemiol Biomarkers Prev 2018; 27(11):1265–74.

6. Mercado C, Zingmond D, Karlan BY, et al. Quality of care in advanced ovarian cancer: the importance of provider specialty. Gynecol Oncol 2010;117(1):18–22.

7. Sullivan MW, Camacho FT, Mills AM, et al. Missing information in statewide and national cancer databases: correlation with health risk factors, geographic disparities, and outcomes. Gynecol Oncol 2019;152(1):119–26.

8. Park J, Blackburn BE, Rowe K, et al. Rural-metropolitan disparities in ovarian cancer survival: a statewide population-based study. Ann Epidemiol 2018;28(6): 377–84.

9. Zahnd WE, Hyon KS, Diaz-Sylvester P, et al. Rural–urban differences in surgical treatment, regional lymph node examination, and survival in endometrial cancer patients. Cancer Causes Control 2018;29(2):221–32.

10. Bristow RE, Chang J, Ziogas A, et al. Spatial analysis of adherence to treatment guidelines for advanced-stage ovarian cancer and the impact of race and socioeconomic status. Gynecol Oncol 2014;134(1):60–7.

11. Gunderson CC, Tergas AI, Fleury AC, et al. Primary uterine cancer in Maryland: impact of distance on access to surgical care at high-volume hospitals. Int J Gynecol Cancer 2013;23(7):1244–51.

12. Gunderson CC, Nugent EK, McMeekin DS, et al. Distance traveled for treatment of cervical cancer: who travels the farthest, and does it impact outcome? Int J Gynecol Cancer 2013;23(6):1099–103.

13. Barrington DA, Dilley SE, Landers EE, et al. Distance from a comprehensive cancer center: a proxy for poor cervical cancer outcomes? Gynecol Oncol 2016; 143(3):617–21.

14. Tan W, Stehman FB, Carter RL. Mortality rates due to gynecologic cancers in New York state by demographic factors and proximity to a Gynecologic Oncology Group member treatment center: 1979-2001. Gynecol Oncol 2009;114(2): 346–52.

15. Benjamin I, Dalton H, Qiu Y, et al. Endometrial cancer surgery in Arizona: a statewide analysis of access to care. Gynecol Oncol 2011;121(1):83–6.

16. Spees LP, Wheeler SB, Varia M, et al. Evaluating the urban-rural paradox: the complicated relationship between distance and the receipt of guideline-concordant care among cervical cancer patients. Gynecol Oncol 2019;152(1): 112–8.

17. Shalowitz DI, Nivasch E, Burger RA, et al. Are patients willing to travel for better ovarian cancer care? Gynecol Oncol 2017. https://doi.org/10.1016/j.ygyno.2017. 10.018.

18. Wright AA, Bohlke K, Armstrong DK, et al. Neoadjuvant chemotherapy for newly diagnosed, advanced ovarian cancer: Society of Gynecologic Oncology and American Society of Clinical Oncology Clinical Practice Guideline. Gynecol Oncol 2016;143(1):3–15.

19. National Comprehensive Cancer Network. NCCN clinical practice guidelines in oncology: cervical cancer version 4.2019. 2019. Available at: https://www.nccn.org/professionals/physician_gls/pdf/cervical.pdf.

20. American College of Obstetricians and Gynecologists' Committee on Practice Bulletins—Gynecology. Practice bulletin No. 174. Obstet Gynecol 2016;128(5):e210–26.

21. National Comprehensive Cancer Network. NCCN clinical practice guidelines in oncology: uterine neoplasms Version 3.2019. 2019. Available at: https://www.nccn.org/professionals/physician_gls/pdf/uterine.pdf.

22. Shalowitz DI, Vinograd AM, Giuntoli RL. Geographic access to gynecologic cancer care in the United States. Gynecol Oncol 2015;138(1):115–20.

23. Stewart SL, Cooney D, Hirsch S, et al. Effect of gynecologic oncologist availability on ovarian cancer mortality. World J Obstet Gynecol 2014;3(2):71.

24. Moss JL, Liu B, Feuer EJ. Urban/rural differences in breast and cervical cancer incidence: the mediating roles of socioeconomic status and provider density. Womens Health Issues 2017;27(6):683–91.

25. Unger JM, Moseley A, Symington B, et al. Geographic distribution and survival outcomes for rural patients with cancer treated in clinical trials. JAMA Netw Open 2018;1(4):e181235.

26. Farley JH, Hines JF, Taylor RR, et al. Equal care ensures equal survival for African-American women with cervical carcinoma. Cancer 2001;91(4):869–73. Available at: http://www.ncbi.nlm.nih.gov/pubmed/11241257. Accessed February 18, 2015.

27. Bristow RE, Palis BE, Chi DS, et al. The National Cancer Database report on advanced-stage epithelial ovarian cancer: impact of hospital surgical case volume on overall survival and surgical treatment paradigm. Gynecol Oncol 2010;118(3):262–7.

28. Fung-Kee-Fung M, Kennedy EB, Biagi J, et al. The optimal organization of gynecologic oncology services: a systematic review. Curr Oncol 2015;22(4):282.

29. Shalowitz DI, Epstein AJ, Ko EM, et al. Non-surgical management of ovarian cancer: prevalence and implications. Gynecol Oncol 2016;142(1). https://doi.org/10.1016/j.ygyno.2016.04.026.

30. Cliby WA, Powell MA, Al-Hammadi N, et al. Ovarian cancer in the United States: contemporary patterns of care associated with improved survival. Gynecol Oncol 2014. https://doi.org/10.1016/j.ygyno.2014.10.023.

31. Tracy R, Nam I, Gruca TS. The influence of visiting consultant clinics on measures of access to cancer care: evidence from the state of Iowa. Health Serv Res 2013;48(5):1719–29.

32. Gruca TS, Nam I, Tracy R. Trends in medical oncology outreach clinics in rural areas. J Oncol Pract 2014;10(5):e313–20.

33. Reade C, Elit L. Trends in gynecologic cancer care in North America. Obstet Gynecol Clin North Am 2012;39(2):107–29.

34. McCluggage WG, Judge MJ, Clarke BA, et al. Data set for reporting of ovary, fallopian tube and primary peritoneal carcinoma: recommendations from the International Collaboration on Cancer Reporting (ICCR). Mod Pathol 2015;28(8):1101–22.

35. Holschneider CH, Petereit DG, Chu C, et al. Brachytherapy: a critical component of primary radiation therapy for cervical cancer. Gynecol Oncol 2019;152(3):540–7.

36. Lakhman Y, D'Anastasi M, Miccò M, et al. Second-opinion interpretations of gynecologic oncologic MRI examinations by sub-specialized radiologists influence patient care. Eur Radiol 2016;26(7):2089–98.
37. Mullen MM, Cripe JC, Thaker PH. Palliative care in gynecologic oncology. Obstet Gynecol Clin North Am 2019;46(1):179–97.
38. Ring KL, Garcia C, Thomas MH, et al. Current and future role of genetic screening in gynecologic malignancies. Am J Obstet Gynecol 2017;217(5):512–21.
39. McKenney KM, Martinez NG, Yee LM. Patient navigation across the spectrum of women's health care in the United States. Am J Obstet Gynecol 2018;218(3):280–6.
40. Shalowitz DI, Cohn DE. Cancer care delivery research in gynecologic oncology. Gynecol Oncol 2018;148(3):445–8.
41. Bashshur RL, Krupinski EA, Weinstein RS, et al. The empirical foundations of telepathology: evidence of feasibility and intermediate effects. Telemed J E Health 2017;23(3):155–91.
42. Bashshur RL, Krupinski EA, Thrall JH, et al. The empirical foundations of teleradiology and related applications: a review of the evidence. Telemed J E Health 2016;22(11):868–98.
43. Cook DA, Sorensen KJ, Wilkinson JM. Value and process of curbside consultations in clinical practice: a grounded theory study. Mayo Clin Proc 2014;89(5):602–14.
44. Association of American Medical Colleges. Project CORE: coordinating optimal referral experiences. 2019. Available at: https://www.aamc.org/initiatives/core2/.
45. Project Echo - The University of New Mexico. Project ECHO model. 2015. Available at: http://echo.unm.edu/about-echo/model/. Accessed June 22, 2019.
46. Atlas I, Granai CO, Gajewski W, et al. Videoconferencing for gynaecological cancer care: an international tumour board. J Telemed Telecare 2000;6(4):242–4. Available at: http://www.ncbi.nlm.nih.gov/pubmed/11027128. Accessed February 27, 2015.
47. Chekerov R, Denkert C, Boehmer D, et al. Online tumor conference in the clinical management of gynecological cancer: experience from a pilot study in Germany. Int J Gynecol Cancer 2008;18(1):1–7.
48. Sabesan S. Medical models of teleoncology: current status and future directions. Asia Pac J Clin Oncol 2014;10(3):200–4.
49. Sabesan S, Simcox K, Marr I. Medical oncology clinics through videoconferencing: an acceptable telehealth model for rural patients and health workers. Intern Med J 2012;42(7):780–5.
50. Mair F, Whitten P, May C, et al. Patients' perceptions of a telemedicine specialty clinic. J Telemed Telecare 2000;6(1):36–40.
51. Kitamura C, Zurawel-Balaura L, Wong RKS. How effective is video consultation in clinical oncology? A systematic review. Curr Oncol 2010;17(3):17–27. Available at: http://www.pubmedcentral.nih.gov/articlerender.fcgi?artid=2880899&tool=pmcentrez&rendertype=abstract. Accessed March 18, 2015.
52. Jue JS, Spector SA, Spector SA. Telemedicine broadening access to care for complex cases. J Surg Res 2017;220:164–70.
53. Lesher AP, Shah SR. Telemedicine in the perioperative experience. Semin Pediatr Surg 2018;27(2):102–6.
54. Afable MK, Gupte G, Simon SR, et al. Innovative use of electronic consultations in preoperative anesthesiology evaluation at VA Medical Centers In New England. Health Aff 2018;37(2):275–82.

55. Shalowitz DI, Epstein AJ, Buckingham L, et al. Survival implications of time to surgical treatment of endometrial cancers. Am J Obstet Gynecol 2017;216(3): 268.e1-18.

56. Marescaux J, Leroy J, Rubino F, et al. Transcontinental robot-assisted remote telesurgery: feasibility and potential applications. Ann Surg 2002;235(4):487–92. Available at: http://www.pubmedcentral.nih.gov/articlerender.fcgi?artid=14224 62&tool=pmcentrez&rendertype=abstract. Accessed February 25, 2015.

57. Perez M, Xu S, Chauhan S, et al. Impact of delay on telesurgical performance: study on the robotic simulator dV-Trainer. Int J Comput Assist Radiol Surg 2016;11(4):581–7.

58. Xu S, Perez M, Yang K, et al. Effect of latency training on surgical performance in simulated robotic telesurgery procedures. Int J Med Robot 2014. https://doi.org/10.1002/rcs.1623.

59. Stark M, Pomati S, D'Ambrosio A, et al. A new telesurgical platform - preliminary clinical results. Minim Invasive Ther Allied Technol 2015;24(1):31–6.

60. Reichenbach M, Frederick T, Cubrich L, et al. Telesurgery with miniature robots to leverage surgical expertise in distributed expeditionary environments. Mil Med 2017;182(S1):316–21.

61. Erridge S, Yeung DKT, Patel HRH, et al. Telementoring of surgeons: a systematic review. Surg Innov 2019;26(1):95–111.

62. Shalowitz DI, Goodwin A, Schoenbachler N. Does surgical treatment of atypical endometrial hyperplasia require referral to a gynecologic oncologist? Am J Obstet Gynecol 2019;220(5):460–4.

63. Gunter RL, Chouinard S, Fernandes-Taylor S, et al. Current use of telemedicine for post-discharge surgical care: a systematic review. J Am Coll Surg 2016; 222(5):915–27.

64. Graetz I, Anderson JN, McKillop CN, et al. Use of a web-based app to improve postoperative outcomes for patients receiving gynecological oncology care: a randomized controlled feasibility trial. Gynecol Oncol 2018;150(2):311–7.

65. Armstrong KA, Coyte PC, Brown M, et al. Effect of home monitoring via mobile app on the number of in-person visits following ambulatory surgery: a randomized clinical trial. JAMA Surg 2017;152(7):622–7.

66. Lu K, Marino NE, Russell D, et al. Use of short message service and smartphone applications in the management of surgical patients: a systematic review. Telemed J E Health 2018;24(6):406–14.

67. Matousek A, Paik K, Winkler E, et al. Community health workers and smartphones for the detection of surgical site infections in rural Haiti: a pilot study. Lancet 2015; 385(Suppl 2):S47.

68. Pathak A, Sharma S, Sharma M, et al. Feasibility of a mobile phone-based surveillance for surgical site infections in rural India. Telemed J E Health 2015;21(11): 946–9.

69. Bednarski BK, Slack RS, Katz M, et al. Assessment of ileostomy output using telemedicine: a feasibility trial. Dis Colon Rectum 2018;61(1):77–83.

70. Nandra K, Koenig G, DelMastro A, et al. Telehealth provides a comprehensive approach to the surgical patient. Am J Surg 2018. https://doi.org/10.1016/j.amjsurg.2018.09.020.

71. Doolittle GC, Spaulding AO. Providing access to oncology care for rural patients via telemedicine. J Oncol Pract 2006;2(5):228–30. Available at: http://www.pubmedcentral.nih.gov/articlerender.fcgi?artid=2793628&tool=pmcentrez&rendertype=abstract. Accessed February 25, 2015.

72. Pathmanathan S, Burgher B, Sabesan S. Is intensive chemotherapy safe for rural cancer patients? Intern Med J 2013;43(6):643–9.
73. Chan BA, Larkins SL, Evans R, et al. Do teleoncology models of care enable safe delivery of chemotherapy in rural towns? Med J Aust 2015;203(10):406.
74. Buchanan AH, Datta SK, Skinner CS, et al. Randomized trial of telegenetics vs. in-person cancer genetic counseling: cost, patient satisfaction and attendance. J Genet Couns 2015;24(6):961–70.
75. Fridriksdottir N, Gunnarsdottir S, Zoëga S, et al. Effects of web-based interventions on cancer patients' symptoms: review of randomized trials. Support Care Cancer 2018;26(2):337–51.
76. Warrington L, Absolom K, Conner M, et al. Electronic systems for patients to report and manage side effects of cancer treatment: systematic review. J Med Internet Res 2019;21(1):e10875.
77. Moradian S, Voelker N, Brown C, et al. Effectiveness of Internet-based interventions in managing chemotherapy-related symptoms in patients with cancer: a systematic literature review. Support Care Cancer 2018;26(2):361–74.
78. Cowan RA, Suidan RS, Andikyan V, et al. Electronic patient-reported outcomes from home in patients recovering from major gynecologic cancer surgery: a prospective study measuring symptoms and health-related quality of life. Gynecol Oncol 2016;143(2):362–6.
79. Judson TJ, Bennett AV, Rogak LJ, et al. Feasibility of long-term patient self-reporting of toxicities from home via the internet during routine chemotherapy. J Clin Oncol 2013;31(20):2580–5.
80. Worster B, Swartz K. Telemedicine and palliative care: an increasing role in supportive oncology. Curr Oncol Rep 2017;19(6):37.
81. Hoek PD, Schers HJ, Bronkhorst EM, et al. The effect of weekly specialist palliative care teleconsultations in patients with advanced cancer –a randomized clinical trial. BMC Med 2017;15(1):119.
82. Natafgi N, Shane DM, Ullrich F, et al. Using tele-emergency to avoid patient transfers in rural emergency departments: an assessment of costs and benefits. J Telemed Telecare 2018;24(3):193–201.
83. Datta NR, Rajasekar D. Improvement of radiotherapy facilities in developing countries: a three-tier system with a teleradiotherapy network. Lancet Oncol 2004;5(11):695–8.
84. Hamilton E, Van Veldhuizen E, Brown A, et al. Telehealth in radiation oncology at the Townsville Cancer Centre: service evaluation and patient satisfaction. Clin Transl Radiat Oncol 2019;15:20–5.
85. Kisling K, Zhang L, Simonds H, et al. Fully automatic treatment planning for external-beam radiation therapy of locally advanced cervical cancer: a tool for low-resource clinics. J Glob Oncol 2019;5:1–9.
86. Sabesan S, Zalcberg J. Telehealth models could be extended to conducting clinical trials-a teletrial approach. Eur J Cancer Care (Engl) 2018;27(2):e12587.
87. Salani R, Khanna N, Frimer M, et al. An update on post-treatment surveillance and diagnosis of recurrence in women with gynecologic malignancies: Society of Gynecologic Oncology (SGO) recommendations. Gynecol Oncol 2017; 146(1):3–10.
88. Doolittle GC, Nelson E-L, Spaulding AO, et al. TeleHospice: a community-engaged model for utilizing mobile tablets to enhance rural hospice care. Am J Hosp Palliat Med 2019;36(9):795–800.
89. Kidd L, Cayless S, Johnston B, et al. Telehealth in palliative care in the UK: a review of the evidence. J Telemed Telecare 2010;16(7):394–402.

90. Shanafelt TD, Dyrbye LN, Sinsky C, et al. Relationship between clerical burden and characteristics of the electronic environment with physician burnout and professional satisfaction. Mayo Clin Proc 2016;91(7):836–48.
91. Armstrong KA, Semple JL, Coyte PC. Replacing ambulatory surgical follow-up visits with mobile app home monitoring: modeling cost-effective scenarios. J Med Internet Res 2014;16(9):e213.
92. Shalowitz DI, Huh WK. Access to gynecologic oncology care and the network adequacy standard. Cancer 2018. https://doi.org/10.1002/cncr.31392.
93. Venkatesh V, Bala H. Technology acceptance model 3 and a research agenda on interventions. Decis Sci 2008;39(2):273–315.

Telemedicine for Family Planning: A Scoping Review

Terri-Ann Thompson, PhD[a],*, Sarita Sonalkar, MD, MPH[b],
Jessica L. Butler, MPH[c], Daniel Grossman, MD[d]

KEYWORDS

- Telemedicine • Telehealth • Family planning • Contraception • Abortion
- Medication abortion

KEY POINTS

- Text messaging may increase knowledge about contraception, but there is limited evidence about its effectiveness to increase uptake among nonusers.
- Text messaging reminders improve continuation among oral contraceptive and injectable users.
- One study indicates that telemedicine provision of contraception uses evidence-based criteria for assessing eligibility, but more research is needed on this model.
- Telemedicine provision of medication abortion has been shown to be equally safe and effective as in-person provision, and some measures of satisfaction are higher with telemedicine.
- Telemedicine provision of medication abortion improved access to early abortion in 1 study in Iowa.

BACKGROUND

Despite significant advances in contraceptive technology and the availability of a nonsurgical option for abortion, the benefits of family planning remain limited by the number of people who can access services. Contributing factors of low family planning use includes inadequate access to contraception and medication abortion, limited user and provider knowledge of family planning methods, inconsistent and/or incorrect use

[a] Ibis Reproductive Health, 2067 Massachusetts Avenue, Suite 320, Cambridge, MA 02140, USA;
[b] Department of Obstetrics and Gynecology, University of Pennsylvania, 1000 Courtyard, 3400 Spruce Street, Philadelphia, PA 19104, USA; [c] The American College of Obstetricians and Gynecologists, 409 12th Street, Southwest, PO Box 96920, Washington, DC 20090-6920, USA;
[d] Department of Obstetrics, Gynecology and Reproductive Sciences, Advancing New Standards in Reproductive Health (ANSIRH), Bixby Center for Global Reproductive Health, University of California San Francisco, 1330 Broadway, Suite 1100, Oakland, CA 94612, USA
* Corresponding author.
E-mail address: tthompson@ibisreproductivehealth.org
Twitter: @DrDGrossman (D.G.)

of contraception, and nonuse of contraception. Efforts to address these factors include significant investments in family planning services through global campaigns such as Family Planning 2020,[1] efforts to create more effective supply chains,[2] and the use of technology to facilitate access to services and information.[3,4]

The World Health Organization defines telemedicine broadly as the

> delivery of health care services, where distance is a critical factor, by all health care professionals using information and communication technologies for the exchange of valid information for diagnosis, treatment and prevention of disease and injuries, research and evaluation, and for the continuing education of health care providers, all in the interests of advancing the health of individuals and their communities.[5]

The use of telemedicine in obstetrics and gynecology has grown substantially in the last decade, with technology being used to counsel patients, consult with specialists, conduct ultrasounds, and manage illnesses during and after pregnancy, such as diabetes and postpartum depression.[6–9] With telemedicine, care may either be delivered to a patient from (1) a remote location virtually and in real time (synchronous delivery) or (2) through static health information generated by health experts offline (asynchronous delivery). In the case of family planning, technology such as mobile phone applications (apps), websites, short message service/text messaging, telephone, and live audiovisual communication has been used to support contraceptive initiation, adherence, and continuation as well as deliver medication abortion services and follow-up to patients.

An assessment of the current use and existing research on telemedicine can help to guide clinicians in adding or testing the feasibility of telemedicine interventions for family planning within current clinical practice, encourage shared lessons across geographic contexts, and highlight spaces where more evidence is needed to reduce barriers to family planning use. Therefore, the aim of this study was to conduct a scoping review to identify and synthesize the evidence on the use of telemedicine for family planning.

METHODS
Protocol and Registration

The protocol for this scoping review was registered with the Open Science Framework and is publicly available.

Scope of Review

This scoping review was designed to map the evidence and highlight key knowledge gaps on the use of mobile phone, online platforms, remote monitoring and care delivery, and virtual visits for family planning. The key questions addressed in this review are:

- KQ1. How has telemedicine been used for family planning?
- KQ2. Who are the targets of telemedicine for family planning?
- KQ3. What outcomes have been assessed for telemedicine for family planning?

We used the PRISMA extension[10] for scoping reviews to guide the review and format for this article.

Eligibility criteria
Eligibility criteria were broadly set to ensure a wide capture of studies that describe and evaluate the use of telecommunications technology for 3 family planning services:

contraception, medication abortion, and remote follow-up after medication abortion. To be included in this review, articles had to be in English, assess patient and/or provider populations, and describe an intervention where technology was used to provide a clinical service. Clinical service encompassed diagnostic, therapeutic, or preventive (including counseling) procedures. Additionally, articles that described peer-to-peer specialty consultations through virtual visits, direct-to-patient virtual visits, remote patient monitoring, mobile health and apps, and health care delivery apps/platforms were included. There were no restrictions placed on the year in which the study was published, the study design, or settings in which telemedicine for family planning was being used.

Search and screening strategy

We adapted a comprehensive set of search terms developed by the authors in collaboration with American College of Gynecologists Resource Center senior medical librarians for a previous systematic review of telehealth interventions for obstetrics and gynecology. A list of the search terms used for one database is included in **Box 1**. A comprehensive literature search was performed for primary literature in

---

Box 1
Index and keyword terms used for one database

1. Telemedicine/or telemedicine.ti,ab. or (interactive adj3 consult$).ti,ab. or (interactive adj3 diagnos$).ti,ab. or (health adj3 mobile).ti,ab. or (mobile adj3 health).ti,ab. or telehealth.ti,ab. or (ehealth or e-health).ti,ab. or (mhealth or m-health).ti,ab. or (telecommunications/and remote.ti,ab.) or remote consultation/or (remote adj3 consult$).ti,ab. or (remote adj3 telecommunication$).ti,ab. or (video adj3 visit$).ti,ab. or (remote adj3 visit$).ti,ab. or (remote adj3 monitor$).ti,ab. or (mobile adj3 app$).ti,ab. or (mobile adj3 media).ti,ab. or (digital adj3 health).ti,ab. or ((smartphone$ or smart phone$) adj3 app$).ti,ab. or smartphone/or mobile applications/or (secure adj3 message$).ti,ab. or wearable$.ti,ab. or (wearable$ adj3 device$).ti,ab. or (patient adj3 generate$ adj3 data).ti,ab. or (distance adj3 health).ti,ab. or (connect$ adj3 health).ti,ab. or (remote.ti,ab. and videoconferencing/) or (remote adj3 videoconferenc$).ti,ab. or telepharmacy.ti,ab. or (telemedicine/and (pharmacy service, hospital/or community pharmacy services/)) or teleradiology/or teleradiology.ti,ab. or ((radiology information systems/or technology, radiologic/) and telemedicine/) or telepathology/or telepathology.ti,ab. or (pathology/and telemedicine/) or in-home.ti,ab. or (wireless adj4 monitor$).ti,ab. or teleultraso$.ti,ab. or tele-ultraso$.ti,ab. or tele-radiology.ti,ab. or tele-pathology.ti,ab. or tele-pharmacy.ti,ab. or tele-medicine.ti,ab. or tele-health.ti,ab. or (virtual adj3 care).ti,ab. or (remote adj3 care).ti,ab. or (digital adj3 technolog$).ti,ab. or (portable adj3 device$).ti,ab. or ((phone or telephone or smartphone or smart phone) adj3 based).ti,ab. or (text adj3 messag$).ti,ab. or ((sms adj3 messag$) or short message service$).ti,ab. or (tablet adj3 app$).ti,ab. or (computers, handheld/and mobile applications/) or (patient adj3 engage$ adj3 app$).ti,ab. or (virtual adj3 consult$).ti,ab. or (virtual adj3 visit$).ti,ab. or (virtual adj3 health$).ti,ab.

2. Obstetrics/or gynecology/or womens health/or women's health services/or exp contraceptive agents, female/or exp contraceptive devices, female/or exp maternal health services/or exp *pregnancy outcome/or exp "Female Urogenital Diseases and Pregnancy Complications"/or exp "diagnostic techniques, obstetrical and gynecological"/or exp gynecologic surgical procedures/or exp obstetric surgical procedures/

3. Family planning.mp. or Family Planning Services/or exp Contraception/or Contraception, postcoital/or Contraception, barrier/or Contraception, behavior/or contracept$.mp. or abortion.mp. or exp Intrauterine devices/or "birth control".mp. or Abortion, Induced/or Abortion, Legal/or (pregnancy adj3 terminat$).mp. or post-abortion.mp.

4. exp contraceptive agents, female/or exp contraceptive devices, female/

Cochrane Library, Cochrane Collaboration Registry of Controlled Trials, EMBASE, PubMed, and MEDLINE. The search was completed in September 2017 and updated in 2018 and July 2019 to capture additional studies published between initiation and completion of this review. The authors conducted abstract and full text review to identify peer-reviewed studies for inclusion. Observational studies (retrospective and prospective), systematic reviews, randomized controlled trials (RCTs), and outcome evaluations of telemedicine for 3 family planning services were included. Qualitative and quantitative studies were included with no restrictions placed on sample size.

A data extraction form, developed by the lead author, included variables aligned with the key research questions. The variables included general information and evaluation (**Table 1**). Extracted data were collected in a table and analyzed by family planning service. Studies were reviewed and findings confirmed by authors. Discrepancies in study inclusion were resolved through discussion among the authors.

RESULTS

A total of 533 studies were eligible for initial review. After excluding duplicates, studies in languages other than English, commentaries, abstract-only publications, case reports/series, and studies that reviewed services other than family planning services, 43 studies were included in this scoping review; 14 studies on contraception, 20 studies on medication abortion, and 9 studies on medication abortion follow-up (**Fig. 1**). Publication years ranged from 2008 to 2019 and included telemedicine services in countries in the very high, high, and medium Human Development Index.[11]

Contraception

Contraception studies included in this review examined technological interventions that could facilitate the initiation and use, adherence, continuation, and provision of a contraceptive method. The majority of studies in this review used mobile apps or text message reminders (n = 12). One study described a telephone intervention and another an online platform for oral contraceptive prescriptions. Studies on contraception were done in the last 10 years, between 2008 and 2019 and mapped to at least 1 contraception outcome. All studies in this review used quantitative methods to assess a range of indicators (**Table 2**).

Initiation and use

Two RCTs piloted programs to increase contraceptive knowledge and facilitate long-acting reversible contraceptive uptake.[12,13] Smith and colleagues' study,[13] based in Cambodia, targeted women seeking safe abortion services. Women were randomized to either a 3-month mobile phone-based intervention—where they received 6 automated, interactive voice messages with counselor phone support (depending on their response to the message) or to a control group receiving standard care, postabortion family planning counseling at the clinic, the offer of a follow-up appointment at the clinic, and contact information for the clinic inclusive of a hotline number operated

Table 1	
List of variables extracted for each family planning service	
General Information	Defined as publication year, geographic location, study type (quantitative or qualitative), telemedicine model, and family planning service
Evaluation	Study design, sample size, outcome, data collection methods, population studied, gestational age

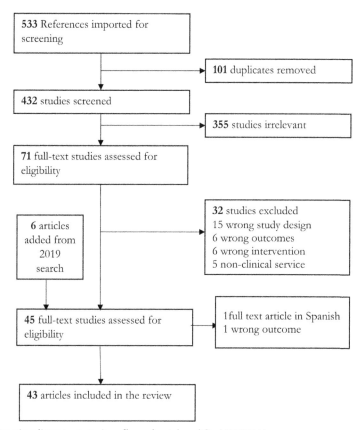

Fig. 1. Scoping literature review flow chart (modified PRISMA).

by the counsellors. Women were contacted at 4 and 12 months to determine if they had initiated and continued use of a contraceptive method, respectively. In Gilliam and colleagues' study,[12] women were randomized to either receive the app and standard of care or just standard of care (described as contraceptive counseling by a clinic counselor followed by a visit with a nurse practitioner to receive [or be prescribed] the contraceptive method of their choice). Those randomized to the intervention arm received a tablet computer with the contraception information app and instructions to use the app for up to 15 minutes. Authors reported a significant increase in contraceptive knowledge among app users,[12] increased interest in the implant as a contraceptive method,[12] and an increase in short-term use of any effective contraceptive method and the use of a long-acting contraceptive method in the longer term.[13]

Two RCTs evaluated the use of a text messaging intervention to increase oral contraceptive knowledge and contraceptive use among young women, ages 13 to 25.[4,14] Educational texts were sent daily for 3[14] and 6 months.[4] The text message intervention was not shown to increase contraceptive initiation; however, modest improvements were observed in oral contraceptive knowledge over time.[4] Two RCTs of text message interventions with young people, 14 to 18 years old, in the United States[15] and 16 to 24 in Tajikistan[16] were included in this review. Both studies showed no impact on condom[15] and contraceptive use,[15,16] or in the acceptability of effective contraception.[16]

Table 2
Summary of studies on telemedicine for contraception

Author, Year, Country	Methods	Objective (s)	Results
Gilliam et al,[12] 2014, United States	RCT of patients, under 30 y, in a Title X clinic (28 intervention and 24 standard care)	Assess the impact of an iOS waiting room app for contraceptive counseling on contraceptive knowledge and uptake	Significantly higher knowledge of contraceptive effectiveness among app users Significantly higher interest in the implant method among app users after the intervention (7.1%–32.1%; $P = .02$) No significant difference in LARC selection between arms (25% vs 20.8%; $P = .72$) Acceptability of app use among staff
Smith et al,[13] 2015, Cambodia	RCT of abortion patients, ≥18 y (249 mobile phone users; 251 standard care)	Assess the effect of a mobile phone-based intervention on postabortion contraception use at 4 and 12 mo	Significantly higher proportion of women in intervention group report effective contraception use at 4 mo (64% vs 46%) A significantly higher proportion of women in intervention group report using a long-acting contraceptive method at 4 and 12 mo (29% vs 9% and 25% vs 12%, respectively)
Stidham Hall et al,[4] 2013, United States	RCT of women ages 13–25 y (337 routine care; 346 routine care plus 6 months of daily educational text messages)	Assess the effect of text message reminders on young women's oral contraceptive knowledge	Oral contraceptive knowledge improved over time for all women Mean knowledge scores were significantly greater among women in the intervention group (intervention [25.5] vs control group [23.7])

Study	Design/Population	Objective	Findings
Chernick et al,[14] 2017, United States	RCT of adolescent (14–19 y) emergency department patients receiving texts for 3 months (50 per arm)	Assess the effect of a text messaging intervention on initiation of contraception	Mobile text messaging intervention was acceptable to users Contraceptive initiation limited; initiated in 12% of adolescents in intervention group vs 22.4% in the control group
Bull et al,[15] 2016, United States	RCT of 8 Boys & Girls Clubs into treatment and control sites (youth, 14–18 y; 317 intervention; 315 standard program)	Assess whether the addition of a text messaging intervention increased the effects of an adolescent pregnancy prevention program	No significant differences in condom and contraceptive use, access to care, or pregnancy prevention Hispanic participants in the intervention condition had significantly fewer pregnancies at follow-up (1.79%) than did those in the control group (6.72%)
McCarthy et al,[16] 2018, Tajikistan	RCT of men and women aged 16–24 y (275 intervention arm, 298 control arm)	Assess the effect of a text messaging intervention on acceptability of effective contraceptive methods and contraceptive use at 4 mo and during the study, service uptake, induced abortion, and unintended pregnancy	There was no evidence of a difference in acceptability between groups. Similarly there was no significant difference in contraceptive use, service uptake, or other secondary or process outcomes. Acceptability of effective contraception significantly increased from baseline to follow-up (2%–65%)
Buchanan et al,[17] 2018, United States	Retrospective cohort study of urban adolescent and young adult women (13–21 y). Sixty-seven participants using DMPA at baseline, followed up 20 mo after the intervention	Assess the long term impact of a 9-mo text message intervention on adherence to effective contraceptive methods	Participants in the intervention were close to 4 times more likely to continue using DMPA or a more efficacious method such as implant or intrauterine device at 20 mo after the intervention (odds ratio, 3.65; 95% confidence interval, 1.26–10.08; $P = .015$)

(continued on next page)

Table 2
(continued)

Author, Year, Country	Methods	Objective (s)	Results
Castano et al,[18] 2012, United States	RCT of young women (13–25 y) choosing OCPs at an urban family planning health center (337 routine care; 346 routine care and daily educational text messages)	Assess whether text messaging intervention affects oral contraceptive pill continuation at 6 mo	Significantly higher proportion of OCP users in the intervention group were still users at 6 mo (64% vs 54%) Continuation on the method lessened once the intervention ended
Trent et al,[19] 2015, United States	RCT of urban adolescent and young adult women (13–21 y) using DMPA (50 per arm)	Determine feasibility and acceptability of text messaging intervention	Text messaging intervention feasible and acceptable as a clinical support tool for urban young women Preliminary evidence for text message reminders improving clinic attendance for first 2 family planning visits. Return for first and second cycles were higher for youth in the intervention group vs those in the control
Hou et al,[20] 2010, United States	RCT of young women, 18–30 y). Pill taking was tracked for 3 mo by an electronic monitoring device with wireless data collection (41 per arm)	Assess whether daily text message reminders can increase oral contraceptive pill adherence	Oral contraceptive pill adherence was not improved with daily text message reminders; no significant difference in mean number of missed pills per cycle between groups
Tsur et al,[21] 2008, United States	RCT of women (16–45 y) using isotretinoin, a treatment for severe acne (50 intervention, 58 control), follow-up at 3 mo	Assess the impact of a text message intervention on increasing contraceptive use	No significant difference in contraceptive use between groups at follow-up (50% intervention and 40% control group were using a contraceptive method at 3 mo)

Thiel et al,[22] 2017, United States	Quasiexperimental study with 365 matched pairs (women 14 y and older)	Determine whether Bedsider text message and e-mail reminders increase family planning contraceptive continuation and appointment rates	No significant difference in timely return for contraceptive injections between groups. No difference in contraceptive coverage between groups
Wilkinson et al,[23] 2017, United States	RCT of women, 13–21 y in an urban adolescent clinic	Assess the feasibility of using text messages to remind adolescents to fulfill their advance emergency contraception prescriptions	Study not powered to assess differences across randomized groups; however, preliminary results show prescription fulfilment following text message reminders. The effect seemed to be additive after each text reminder
Zuniga et al,[24] 2018, United States	Assessment of 9 online platforms that prescribe hormonal contraceptives across various states in the United States	Compare prescribing processes and policies of online platforms in the United States and assess whether online prescribers are providing evidence-based care	Variation in the all parts of the prescribing process (how the patient provides information, who reviews patient information to decide eligibility, and screening for contraindications) across platforms. Online prescription platforms serve limited geographic areas. Variation in the range of contraceptive methods offered, fees for services, and policies around age restrictions for contraceptives

Abbreviations: DMPA, depot medroxyprogesterone acetate; LARC, long-acting reversible contraceptive; OCP, oral contraceptive pill.

Continuation

A retrospective cohort study[17] and 2 RCTs[18,19] show a beneficial effect of daily inter-active text message reminders on oral contraceptive and injectable contraceptive continuation. Participants were followed over time for a period of 6[18] and 20 months.[17] Results from the larger RCT showed that the intervention group had significantly higher continuation rates with no difference by age, history of oral contraceptive use, or race.[18] Findings from the injectable contraceptive studies found that interven-tion participants returned sooner after a scheduled appointment for the first cycle[19] and were 3.65 times more likely to continue use of injectables or a more efficacious method at the 20-month postintervention evaluation.[17]

Adherence

Two RCTs[20,21] and 1 quasiexperimental study[22] aimed to understand the impact of daily text message/email reminders on oral contraceptive pill adherence. Results showed no effect of daily text message/email reminders on missed pills as assessed by electronic medication monitoring,[20] no effect on contraceptive use among women using isotretinoin,[21] and no effect on timely return for contraceptive refills and injec-tions.[22] Results from a randomized pilot study of young women who received text messages as a reminder to fulfill their advance emergency contraceptive prescriptions showed a potential temporal effect that seemed to be additive after each text reminder.[23]

Provision

Finally, Zuniga and colleagues[24] compared the prescribing processes and policies of online platforms that prescribe hormonal contraceptives to patients in the United States and assessed whether these platforms were providing evidence-based care based on the 2016 US Medical Eligibility Criteria for Contraceptive Use.[25] To use these platforms, a patient provides relevant information to a health care provider through a remote web portal or sometimes through a synchronous video interaction. The pro-vider reviews the health information, prescribes an appropriate contraceptive method, and sends the contraceptive in the mail or sends a prescription to the patient's phar-macy. The platforms varied in the range of methods offered, fees for services, policies related to age restrictions, and prescribing processes; however, in general the online platforms appropriately screened potential users according to the US Medical Eligi-bility Criteria for Contraceptive Use.

Telemedicine Provision of Medication Abortion

Medication abortion involves the use of mifepristone together with misoprostol or misoprostol alone to terminate a pregnancy. Telemedicine for the provision of medi-cation abortion, defined as the use of technology to provide or facilitate the safe use of abortion pills, has been in use since 2005.[26] Its use has primarily been in settings where access to abortion is legally restricted or because in-person administration of mifepristone is required. Studies included in this review fall into 2 broad categories: telemedicine as part of the health care delivery system and telemedicine as a means to support or facilitate the use of medication abortion—via user-centered gesta-tional age dating, guidance for at-home use of the medications, or reducing wait times. Studies used both qualitative and quantitative methods, and about half (n = 11) analyzed data retrospectively. Finally, all studies on the use of telemedicine to deliver medication abortion used the combined mifepristone-misoprostol regimen (**Table 3**).

Table 3
Summary of studies on telemedicine for medication abortion and medication abortion follow-up

Author, Year, Country	Methods	Objectives	Results
Aiken et al,[27] 2017, Republic of Ireland and northern Ireland	Retrospective, population based analysis of 1000 women (<20–≥45 y) who self-sourced medical abortion (up to 9 wk gestation) during a 3-year period	Assess the safety and effectiveness of medical abortion through online provision	Overall, 95% reported successful termination of pregnancy without surgical intervention. Eighty-seven women reported seeking medical attention based on symptoms of the medical abortion. No deaths were reported.
Gomperts et al,[28] 2012, multi-country	Retrospective study of 2320 women (16–49 y) who self-sourced medical abortion during a 1-year period	Assess surgical intervention rates across regions for women getting a medical abortion through online provision	There are regional differences in rates of surgical intervention after a medical abortion through online provision; high rates were found in Eastern Europe (14.8%), Latin America (14.4%), and Asia/Oceania (11%). Lower rates were found in Western Europe (5.8%), the Middle East (4.7%), and Africa (6.1%). Clinical practice and guidelines on incomplete abortion rather than complications may explain observed differences. Rate of surgical intervention increased with gestational age. Surgical intervention influenced women's views on the acceptability of the telemedicine provision model.

(continued on next page)

Table 3
(continued)

Author, Year, Country	Methods	Objectives	Results
Gomperts et al,[29] 2014, Brazil	Retrospective study of 370 women (16–49 y) of varying gestational ages (<9 wk to >13 wk) during a year	Assess the safety and effectiveness of medical abortion through online provision	Medical abortion through online provision is effective across gestational ages. Although ongoing pregnancy increases with increasing gestational ages (1.9% for pregnancies at 9 wk, 1.4% for pregnancies 10–12 wk, and 6.9% with pregnancies of 13 wk or more), the difference is nonsignificant. Significant difference in surgical intervention rates (19.3% at <9 wk, 15.5% at 11–12 wk, and 44.8% at >13 wk).
Gomperts et al,[30] 2008, multi-country	Retrospective study of 484 women (15–46 y) ≤9 wk gestation from April to December 2006	Assess the effectiveness and acceptability of medical abortion through online provision	Most (95%) women study found online provision of medical abortion acceptable. <2% of women reported a continuing pregnancy. A 6.8% curettage/vacuum aspiration rate for incomplete termination of pregnancy observed.
Les et al,[31] 2017, Hungary	Retrospective study of 136 women (≤19–≥41 y) over a 5-year period	Assess the safety and acceptability of medical abortion through online provision	Of the 59 women who had a medical abortion, 5 (8.5%) had a surgical intervention. All women who completed the follow-up survey found online provision of medical abortion acceptable.

Hyland et al,[32] 2018, Australia	Retrospective study of 965 women (14–49 y) <8 wk gestation who received services between June 2015 and December 2016	Assess the safety, effectiveness, and acceptability of at-home telemedicine for medication abortion	Nearly all women (97%) indicate the at-home-telemedicine model was acceptable. At-home telemedicine model for medication abortion is effective; 96% of women who had a medical abortion were able to terminate the pregnancy without surgical intervention and 95% had no face-to-face clinical encounter after the medication abortion.
Raymond et al,[33] 2019, United States	Prospective study of 248 women (15–45 y) who received medication abortion packages, across 5 states, from May 2016 and December 2018 Women completing medication abortion using this model were ≤10 wk gestation	Assess the safety, effectiveness, feasibility, and acceptability of at-home telemedicine for medication abortion	64% of women who received medication abortion packages reported being satisfied with the service. Among women who provided abortion outcomes, 93% reported a complete abortion without surgical intervention. Among women who provided follow-up data, reports of clinically adverse events was low: <1% reported hospitalization or excessive bleeding. But 12% had an unscheduled clinical encounter, 50% of which resulted in no treatment.

(continued on next page)

Table 3
(continued)

Author, Year, Country	Methods	Objectives	Results
Endler et al,[34] 2019, Poland	Retrospective population-based analysis of 615 women (16–56 y) from June to December 2016	Assess the safety and acceptability of online provision of medical abortion	Medical abortion through online provision at >9 wk of gestation is associated with higher risk of same-day or day after clinical visits for concerns related to the procedure (11.7% for 9–11 wk and 22.5% for >11–14 wk). Self-reported rates of heavy bleeding, low satisfaction, or unmet expectations with medical abortion do not increase with gestational age.
Wiebe,[35] 2014, Canada	Retrospective chart review of women who completed a medical abortion from May 2012 and May 2013	To pilot and assess feasibility of an at-home telemedicine model for medical abortion	Telemedicine seems to be feasible in this geographic setting. In the launch year, 11 women had a medical abortion; 8 completed with no intervention, only 1 required surgical intervention.
Aiken et al,[42] 2017, Republic of Ireland	Retrospective, population based analysis of 5650 women (<20–≥45 y) who self-sourced medical abortion during a 5 year period	Assess the characteristics and experience of women getting a medical abortion through online provision	High levels of satisfaction with online provision of medical abortion; 98% would recommend it to others in a similar situation and 97% felt they made the right choice. Women report feeling serious mental stress owing to the pregnancy and an inability to travel abroad to access abortion services. 70% reported feeling relieved right after completing the medical abortion.

	Study design	Objective	Findings/Conclusions
Grossman & Grindlay[36] 2017, United States	Retrospective cohort study of 8765 telemedicine and 10,405 in-person medical abortions performed over a 7-year period; women ≤9 wk gestation	Assess the safety of clinic-to-clinic telemedicine provision of medical abortion (as compared with in person)	Adverse events are rare with medical abortion; no deaths reported. <1% of telemedicine and in-person patients had any adverse event.
Grossman et al,[37] 2011, United States	Prospective cohort study of 449 women (18–45 y) who obtained medical abortion through an in-person visit or via clinic-to-clinic telemedicine over a year (2008–2009)	Assess the safety and acceptability of a clinic-to-clinic telemedicine model for medical abortion	Clinic-to-clinic telemedicine for medical abortion is safe; 99% abortion completion for telemedicine patients and 97% for in-person patients. No significant difference in prevalence of adverse events reported during the study period among telemedicine patients compared with in-person patients/ Ninety-one percent of participants were satisfied with their abortion.
Kohn et al,[38] 2019, United States	Retrospective cohort of 738 telemedicine and 5214 in-person medical abortions performed during a year (2017–2018); gestational age of women (≤19–≥40 y) was ≤7 wk	Assess the safety and effectiveness of clinic-to-clinic telemedicine provision of medical abortion (as compared with in-person)	Adverse events are rare with medical abortion; no deaths reported. <1% of telemedicine and in-person patients had an adverse event. Ongoing pregnancy (0.5% vs 1.8%) and aspiration procedures (1.4% vs 4.5%) were less common among telemedicine patients.

(continued on next page)

Table 3
(continued)

Author, Year, Country	Methods	Objectives	Results
Grindlay et al,[39] 2013, United States	Qualitative study of providers and patients (<25 y) in Iowa (25 telemedicine patients, 5 in-person patients, and 15 clinic staff)	Assess acceptability of clinic-to-clinic telemedicine model	Telemedicine highly acceptable to patients and providers. Patients were positive or indifferent about having a conversation in person with the doctor. Several benefits of telemedicine were cited, including decreased travel for patients and providers and more availability of locations and appointment times in comparison with in-person service.
Grindlay & Grossman,[40] 2017, United States	Qualitative study of providers in Alaska (8 providers and staff)	Assess acceptability and impact of clinic-to-clinic telemedicine model on clinic	Integration of clinic-to-clinic telemedicine into standard practice is feasible; integrating new technology into clinic operations was easy, minimal impact on clinic flow, same overall processes as in person. Increases ability to provide patient-centered care; participants able to be seen sooner, closer to home, and have more options in abortion procedure type.

Source	Population/Study design	Objective	Findings
Grossman et al,[3] 2013, United States	Impact evaluation to capture changes in access (distance from patient residential zip code to clinic and closest clinic providing surgical abortion) for all abortion encounters (women 15–44 y) (n = 17,956) 2 y before and after the introduction of a clinic-to-clinic telemedicine model	Assess the effect of a clinic-to-clinic telemedicine model for medical abortion on service delivery in a clinic system in Iowa	Clinic patients had increased odds of obtaining both medical abortion and abortion before 13 wks gestation after telemedicine was introduced, with adjustment for other factors. Women living >50 miles from the nearest clinic offering surgical abortion were more likely to obtain an abortion after telemedicine introduction.
Momberg et al,[43] 2016, South Africa	Observational study of 78 women (18–42 y) seeking an abortion at 2 health care clinics	Assess acceptability of and ability to use an online gestational age calculator to assess eligibility for medical abortion in a nonclinical setting	The online gestational age calculator was considered easy to use, accurate, and helpful by most (86%–94%) participants. On average women overestimated their gestational age by 0.5 d (standard deviation,14.5); not clinically significant.
Constant et al,[44] 2014, South Africa	RCT of women (>18 y) undergoing early medical abortion (standard of care only, n = 235; standard of care + messaging, n = 234)	Assess the impact of automated text messages on anxiety and emotional discomfort, as well as feelings of preparedness among medical abortion seekers	Automated text messages significantly reduced emotional stress and anxiety between baseline and follow-up. Women in the intervention group reported feeling more prepared for bleeding, pain, and side effects associated with medical abortion. Women in the intervention group found text messages highly acceptable and would recommend the messages to a friend.

(continued on next page)

Table 3
(continued)

Author, Year, Country	Methods	Objectives	Results
de Tolly & Constant,[45] 2014, South Africa	RCT of women (>18 y) undergoing early medical abortion (standard of care only, n = 235; standard of care + messaging, n = 234	Assess the feasibility and efficacy of automated text messages	Text messages were highly acceptable and considered a valid form of coaching through the medical abortion process. Women were able to complete a self-assessment questionnaire via mobile phone if given a short training session.
Ehrenreich et al,[47] 2019, United States	Qualitative study with 18 women (19–40 y) who used telemedicine to attend state mandated information visits	Assess patient experience using telemedicine to attend state-mandated information visits	Telemedicine is acceptable as a mode for attending state mandated information visits; technology was easy to use, nurse was attentive to emotions over video. Telemedicine alleviates cost, travel, and time burdens associated with attending 2 in-person visits.
Bracken et al,[48] 2014, United Kingdom	RCT of 999 women (≥16 y) getting remote follow-up (pregnancy test, standardized symptom survey administered via online, text message, or telephone) or to clinic based follow-up with ultrasound at 1 wk; women were ≤63 d of gestation	Assess the effectiveness and feasibility of remote communication technologies to increase follow-up after early medical abortion	Follow-up rate did not differ by group (clinic-based, 73% vs remote, 69%; risk ratio, 1.0; 95% confidence interval, 0.9–1.2). Most women found this follow-up method acceptable, although there was a preference for follow-up by phone or text message in the future. Women in the clinic-based group were 1.9 times more likely to receive some type of additional medical abortion-related care than women in the remote group (risk ratio, 1.875; 95% confidence interval, 1.15–3.06).

Ngoc et al,[49] 2014, Vietnam	RCT of 1433 women (15–46 y) seeking early medical abortion at 4 hospitals getting clinic or phone follow-up; women were ≤63 d of gestation	Assess the effectiveness and feasibility of phone follow-up after early medical abortion	Phone follow-up was highly effective in screening for ongoing pregnancy with a sensitivity and specificity of 92.8% and 90.6%, respectively. The rate of ongoing pregnancy was not significantly different between the 2 groups. 85% of women in the phone group did not need an additional clinic visit.
Platais et al,[50] 2015, Moldova and Uzbekistan	RCT of 2400 women (16–49 y) receiving a medical abortion at ≤63 d gestation (n = 1200 telephone; n = 1200 for clinic follow-up)	Assess the feasibility and acceptability of telephone follow-up combined with a semiquantitative pregnancy test and standard checklist for medical abortion follow-up	Majority of women were successfully contacted by phone (98%). Ongoing pregnancy rate was similar in both groups (0.4%–0.6%), and the semiquantitative pregnancy test identified all ongoing pregnancies in the phone follow-up group. 7% of women in the telephone arm had a clinic follow-up. Women in the phone group found the test and checklist easy to use, and most (76.1%) preferred phone follow-up in the future.

(continued on next page)

Table 3
(continued)

Author, Year, Country	Methods	Objectives	Results
Chen et al,[51] 2016, United States	Retrospective chart review of medical abortions provided over a 3-year period (105 office follow-up; 71 telephone follow-up); women were between 16 and 45 y	Comparing lost to follow-up, abortion completion, and staff effort for medical abortion follow-up by office visit or telephone	Proportion lost to follow-up was similar in both groups. Abortion completion was similar between both groups (94.3% office follow-up vs 92.5% telephone follow-up). Staff made >1 phone call to 43.9% and 69.4% of women at weeks 1 and 4, respectively, and rescheduled 15% of office follow-up visits.
Michie & Cameron,[52] 2014, United Kingdom	A retrospective database review of 1084 women (16–46 y) at a hospital abortion service who had a medical abortion (≤9 wk)	Assess the success of telephone follow-up plus a self-performed LSUP test, in screening for ongoing pregnancies	656 women were successfully contacted, of which 87% screened negative for ongoing pregnancies and 13% screened positive. Only 3 ongoing pregnancies occurred in the 13% of women who screened positive. The sensitivity of telephone follow-up with LSUP to detect ongoing pregnancy was 100% and the specificity was 88%. The negative predictive value was 100%, and the positive predictive value, 3.6%.

| Cameron et al,[53] 2012, Scotland | Retrospective chart review of 476 women (16–46 y) who had telephone follow-up between May 2010 and February 2011 and a prospective study of 75 women after a medical abortion | Assess abortion completion and patient acceptability of telephone follow-up for medical abortion | Telephone follow-up was acceptable; with 100% of surveyed women reporting they would recommend to a friend. 472 women were successfully contacted, of which 60 screened positive for ongoing pregnancy, 3 of whom had ongoing pregnancies, and 1 woman falsely screened negative. The sensitivity of the telephone follow-up was 75%, and specificity was 86%. The negative predictive value was 99.7%, and positive predictive value was 5%. |
| McKay & Rutherford,[54] 2013, United Kingdom | Prospective study of 220 women (<63 d gestation) whose medical abortions were performed at home from September 2009 to October 2010 | Assess the success and acceptability of clinical telephone follow-up for medical abortion | The majority of women were successfully contacted. 3.6% of all medical abortions with clinical telephone follow-up required surgical intervention. Among survey respondents, acceptability of clinical telephone follow-up was high with 95% feeling like they felt prepared for side effects of medical abortion. |

(continued on next page)

Table 3
(continued)

Author, Year, Country	Methods	Objectives	Results
Anger et al,[55] 2019, Mexico	Prospective study of 163 women (14–41 y) who had a medical abortion up to 70 d gestation	Feasibility of an interactive voice response call-in system and at home MLPT for medical abortion follow-up	10 women who reported MLPT results to the interactive voice response system needed clinical evaluation. Ongoing pregnancy was ruled out for 93% of women who reported MLPT results. Among women who had medical abortions after 63 d, MPLT accurately ruled out ongoing pregnancy for 91%.
Perriera et al,[56] 2010, United States	Prospective study of 139 women (18–41 y) up to 63 d of gestation who received a medical abortion	Assess the feasibility of telephone follow-up combined with high sensitivity urine pregnancy test as a method of follow-up to medical abortion	135 women completed follow-up. 26 women were evaluated for a positive or inconclusive pregnancy test. None had a gestational sac or continuing pregnancy. There were 4 continuing pregnancies, 1 before phone call, 2 at a follow-up visit after phone call, and 1 at an interim visit before phone call. The sensitivity of telephone follow-up was 100%, specificity of 86.3%. The negative predictive value was 100% and positive predictive value was 18.2%.

Abbreviations: LSUP, low-sensitivity urine pregnancy; MLPT, multilevel pregnancy test.

Telemedicine as part of the health care delivery system
Direct-to-patient telemedicine models involve the use of telecommunications technology to provide access to the service outside of a clinic setting. Studies that met inclusion criteria featured synchronous and asynchronous models. Patients consult with a provider via a telephone or videoconference. If eligible, the patient is mailed the medications or a prescription is sent to a local pharmacy. After taking the medications, the patient gets follow-up tests and a follow-up consultation with a provider by telephone or videoconference to assess abortion completeness. In contexts where abortion is illegal or highly restricted, patients may access abortion pills through an online platform. Patients complete a consultation form which includes information on pregnancy duration—based on last menstrual period or ultrasound examination—age, pregnancy history, medication history, contraceptive use, and any diseases or allergies. After a review of the medical information and if the clinical criteria are met, the patient is sent a package with the medications along with instructions on its use and support via a helpdesk during and after the abortion process.

Ten studies assessed the safety, effectiveness, and acceptability/satisfaction of direct-to-patient telemedicine models.[27–35] Studies were conducted in very high, high, and medium Human Development Index countries. Seven of the 10 studies assessed the online platform provision of medication abortion pills. Sample sizes for the studies ranged from 11 to 1100. Assessments of effectiveness, safety, and acceptability and satisfaction are captured solely among patients of the telemedicine model. Furthermore, acceptability was only measured from the perspective of the patient. Finally, the direct-to-patient telemedicine model was reported as feasible in a few studies, however, there were no explicit feasibility studies conducted.[33–35]

In the clinic-to-clinic telemedicine model, a patient seeking medication abortion meets with staff in a clinic to obtain a medical history and assess gestational age by ultrasound examination and vital signs. Once complete, the patient meets with a clinician off site via a secure teleconference platform to review their medical history and clinical evaluation, confirm eligibility for the service, and discuss the treatment. If eligible, the patient is provided with the medications and given instructions about taking the misoprostol. Guidance around what to expect during the abortion procedure, warning signs, and a follow-up plan to confirm medication abortion completion is also provided.

Five studies (all conducted in the United States) assessed the safety, effectiveness, and acceptability and satisfaction of clinic-to-clinic models.[36–40] Studies that focused on safety and effectiveness as their primary outcomes used a comparison group design. Three studies were prospective, and the remainder were retrospective reviews. The 2 qualitative studies included in this review examined the experience of patients and providers with the clinic-to-clinic telemedicine model—both the acceptability of the model as well as the impact on services. One study evaluated changes in service delivery statistics in the 2-year period before and after telemedicine was introduced in the clinic system.[3]

Safety and Effectiveness

In 2019, Endler and colleagues,[41] conducted a systematic review of telemedicine for medication abortion (direct-to-patient and clinic-to-clinic models). This review includes several of the articles in our study[27–33,36,37,39,40,42] and concludes that both the clinic-to-clinic and direct-to-patient models are effective and safe. Abortion completion (defined as lack of surgical intervention following the medication abortion), ranged from 98.1% to 100.0% for pregnancies less than 10 weeks gestation age. For direct-to-patient models, where abortion completion was assessed via self-assessment, abortion completion ranged from 76.9% to 96.4%.[27–34] Rates of surgical evacuation after abortion ranged from 0.9% to 19.3%, with 1 study reporting that the higher rate was reflective of clinical practices and guidelines related to incomplete abortion within the geographic context, with a bias toward surgery for complications that may not justify the intervention.[30] The proportion who reported a continuing pregnancy after a medication abortion seemed to increase with gestational ages greater than 10 weeks. Reports from 1 study show continuing pregnancy rates ranging from 1.4% at 10 to 12 weeks to 6.9% at 13 weeks or more.[29] The proportion requiring surgical evacuation increased with gestational age, with 1 study reporting an incidence of 44.8% among participants at more than 13 weeks gestation.[29] Three studies in the systematic review reported on the proportion of women with clinically significant adverse events, defined as death, hospitalization, surgery, blood transfusion, or emergency department visit where treatment was given.[27,32,36] All studies assessed safety among women using medication abortion at less than 10 weeks gestation. Proportion of patients requiring blood transfusion were less than 1%, whereas the proportions of patients requiring hospital admission ranged from 0.07% to 2.80%.[32,36] One study compared safety-related outcomes between women having a medication abortion through telemedicine versus in person at a clinic in Iowa. This retrospective cohort study, with close to 20,000 women over a 7-year period, showed that less than 1% of patients in both the telemedicine and in-person clinic models experienced a clinically adverse event.[36] No deaths were reported in any of the studies. The study concluded that the clinic-to-clinic telemedicine model was noninferior to in-person provision of medication abortion with regard to safety.

Three studies released in 2019 support the findings of this systematic review.[33,34,38] A retrospective cohort study of the clinic-to-clinic model with women presenting at 26 health centers across 4 states (Alaska, Idaho, Nevada, and Washington), found that the proportions of ongoing pregnancy and aspiration procedures among telemedicine and in-person patients were small, less than 2% for ongoing pregnancies and 5% for aspiration procedures.[38] Results from the direct-to-patient models, which included only patients less than 10 weeks gestation, reported that 93%[33] to 97%[34] had a complete abortion. Among women having a medication abortion from 11 to 14 weeks gestation, the proportion of patients requiring hospital admission for concerns related to the treatment was 22.5%.[34]

Acceptability/ Satisfaction

Four of the 10 studies of direct-to-patient telemedicine assessed satisfaction and acceptability.[32–34,42] Acceptability was most often captured through 2 questions: whether the patient would recommend the service to others in a similar situation and overall satisfaction with the service. Less commonly asked of patients is whether they felt the service was the right personal choice for them[42] or valued aspects of the service.[33] Across all studies, acceptability of the telemedicine model was high.

Findings on the acceptability of the clinic-to-clinic telemedicine model comes from 1 prospective study[37] and 2 qualitative studies.[39,40] Results of the prospective study suggest that the majority of patients were satisfied with their abortion and that telemedicine patients were more likely to recommend the service to a friend as compared with in-person patients. That said, about one-quarter of telemedicine patients indicated that they would have preferred to be in the same room as the provider if that had been possible. Younger, nulliparous, and patients with less than a grade 12 education were more likely to report a preference for being in the same room as the provider. Qualitative findings on acceptability from the patient and provider perspective align with quantitative findings. With regard to impact on the clinic, findings from the qualitative studies noted several benefits of the clinic-to-clinic model, including an increase in the number of appointment days and times they could offer to patients, greater availability of locations, and decreased travel times for patients and providers.

Access

Last, Grossman and colleagues[3] evaluated changes in service delivery statistics of 1 clinic system in Iowa following the implementation of a clinic-to-clinic telemedicine model. The pre–post intervention study found that telemedicine was associated with an increase in the probability of a patient receiving a medication abortion and of undergoing a first trimester abortion, as well as a small decrease in travel distance to the clinic. These results suggest that telemedicine provision of medication abortion improves access to early abortion.

Facilitators for medication abortion

Four studies assessed the use of technology to support patients having a medication abortion. Three were conducted in South Africa. They examined an online self-assessment of gestational age[43] and a mobile phone intervention to support patients through medication abortion.[44,45] Studies on the mobile intervention were RCTs aimed at evaluating the acceptability, feasibility, and impact of receiving automated text messages on the symptoms to expect during a medication abortion. The mobile phones coached women through the medication abortion via automated text messages (medication reminder, symptoms, and warning signs) to assess abortion completion, and provide family planning information. The automated text messages were found to be highly acceptable with 98% of those randomized to receive them reporting that the messages helped them through the medication abortion and 99% stating that they would recommend the messages to a friend having the same procedure. Women in the intervention group also reported feeling more prepared for the bleeding and side effects associated with the medication abortion and that they experienced less emotional stress and a decrease in anxiety between baseline and follow-up. A pilot study of 78 women in 2 health centers explored the feasibility and acceptability of an online self-assessment tool for gestational age. They found that women overestimated their gestational age by 0.5 days when compared with ultrasound gestational age, a nonclinically significant difference.[43]

The final study examines the use of telemedicine for state-mandated abortion consent. In 27 states of the United States, patients seeking abortion are required to go through a state-mandated informed consent process and then wait a minimum amount of time before undergoing abortion, most commonly 24 hours.[46] The Planned Parenthood affiliate in Utah, where patients must wait 72 hours, began offering informed consent visits by videoconference in 2015. A qualitative study found that this telemedicine model was feasible and acceptable to patients and helped to decrease the logistical and financial obstacles associated with the mandatory delay requirement.[47]

Remote Follow-Up After Medication Abortion

Studies of remote follow-up after medication abortion involved technology (text message, telephone, or online assessments) paired with a home pregnancy test. Three RCTs explored the efficacy and feasibility of using text, online completion of a symptom questionnaire, or telephone as compared with clinic-based follow-up to confirm abortion completion.[48–50] Follow-up, as defined by rates of complications and ongoing pregnancy, did not differ by group. Three retrospective reviews[51–53] and 3 prospective studies[54–56] of women receiving telephone follow-up after a medication abortion, reported low rates of ongoing pregnancy (<8%). The sensitivity of telephone follow-up ranged from 75%[53] to 100%[56] and specificity from 86%[53] to 88%.[52] Importantly, all 9 studies were done with women at less than or equal to 70 days gestation.

Discussion

Findings from this scoping review suggest several factors that could facilitate the uptake of telemedicine for family planning into standard of practice. First, telemedicine has been effectively used in contraception, medication abortion careand follow-up, and in a mix of very high, high, and medium Human Development Index countries. Second, telemedicine models that use mobile phones with an app or text messaging intervention can be used to decrease emotional stress and help contraception and abortion patients to feel more supported. Third, findings show that telemedicine for medication abortion services is safe, effective, highly acceptable and feasible for patients and providers to integrate into care.

Although there are hundreds of apps that provide sexual and reproductive health information, evaluations of these apps have focused on accuracy and comprehensiveness of information and the features and functionality.[57,58] Our review found no evaluations of sexual and reproductive health apps that assessed knowledge translation as it pertains to contraceptive use, continuation, or translation to better contraceptive counseling practices among family planning providers. The positive effects seen in the study by Gilliam and colleagues[12] suggests that the pairing of an informational app with a provider visit may be better at initiating contraceptive use than having potential users' review and process contraceptive information independently. Presently, evidence for improved initiation and continuation is limited and there is no existing evidence that patient prompts through apps, text messages, or emails lead to better adherence with contraceptive methods. Further, few sexual and reproductive health apps have been found to be accurate, to provide comprehensive contraceptive information, to be developed by reproductive health experts, to cite information from a credible public health source, or advocate for behavior change. These findings, in addition to the lack of regulation of these information apps, makes it difficult to know if and how to incorporate them into clinical practice.

In this review, we identified only 1 study that explored the quality of care provided through online contraception provision platforms. Although there was a wider array of evidence available for medication abortion (ie, safety, effectiveness, acceptability, access, support), the body of evidence was limited by the number of studies available, inclusion of a comparison group, use of convenience samples, use of self-report data, small sample sizes, and high loss to follow-up (for some studies, loss to follow-up was as high as 45%).[30] None of the evaluations of direct-to-patient models included a control group, which is often not feasible in legally restricted settings. More research is needed to reinforce the evidence on medication abortion safety and effectiveness, especially for the direct-to-patient models.

To ensure further adoption of telemedicine into family planning care, a few barriers must be removed. Implementing telemedicine services may be challenging for clinics with limited funds for start-up costs, with low computer or eHealth literacy, and with inadequate connectivity and/or technology infrastructure. However, findings from a systematic review of the use of telemedicine in various medical specialties across 114 countries found that telemedicine could be successfully delivered in settings with limited bandwidth through asynchronous delivery models via email services or static websites.[59] This simple and low-cost solution may be an initial adoption strategy as we work to bolster technology infrastructure and support across health clinics.

Telemedicine's relative newness and variety of applications can also make reimbursement challenging. As an example, some insurance programs in the United States limit the types of providers and services that can be reimbursed for telemedicine or prioritize reimbursement for telemedicine services provided in rural or underserved areas versus urban areas.[60] Finally, the adoption of telemedicine may be limited based on restrictions placed on the family planning service itself. In the United States, strict restrictions on dispensing mifepristone allows for only 1 telemedicine model for medication abortion, the clinic-to-clinic model,[61] which is currently banned in 17 states.[62] Other restrictions include increased requirements to ensure patient security and privacy.

There are a few limitations of this study. The scoping review was limited to telemedicine interventions that have been evaluated and peer reviewed. Therefore, this review may have failed to capture some telemedicine for family planning models or unpublished studies. Further, only English language studies were included in this review. Finally, this review does not incorporate a critical appraisal of the evidence on telemedicine for family planning.

SUMMARY

Telemedicine has the potential to increase access to and quality of use of family planning. In particular, text message reminder apps seem to increase contraceptive method continuation, and preliminary evidence suggests that mobile telemedicine platforms may safely screen potential users for contraceptive eligibility. More research is needed on telemedicine provision of contraception. Although the evidence base is solid for telemedicine provision of medication abortion, more research is needed in particular on direct-to-patient models of care.

DISCLOSURE

Dr D. Grossman has received consulting payments from Planned Parenthood Federation of America for work related to telemedicine for medication abortion.

REFERENCES

1. FP2020 Catalyzing Collaboration 2017-2018. Available at: http://progress.familyplanning2020.org/. Accessed July 10, 2019.
2. World Health Organization. Family Planning Evidence brief: ensuring contraceptive security through effective supply chains. Available at: https://www.who.int/reproductivehealth/publications/family_planning/contraceptive-security-supply-chains/en/. Accessed July 10, 2019.
3. Grossman D, Grindlay K, Buchacker T, et al. Changes in service delivery patterns after introduction of telemedicine provision of medical abortion in Iowa. Am J Public Health 2013;103:73–8.
4. Stidham Hall K, Westhoff CL, Castano PM. The impact of an educational text message intervention on young urban women's knowledge of oral contraception. Contraception 2013;87(4):449–54.
5. World Health Organization. A health telematics policy in support of WHO's Health-For-All strategy for global health development: report of the WHO group consultation on health telematics. Geneva (Switzerland): World Health Organization; 1998.
6. Odibo IN, Wendel PJ, Magann EF. Telemedicine in obstetrics. Clin Obstet Gynecol 2013;56(3):422–33.

7. Magann EF, McKelvey SS, Hitt WC, et al. The use of telemedicine in obstetrics: a review of the literature. Obstet Gynecol Surv 2011;66(3):170–8.
8. Long MC, Angtuaco T, Lowery C. Ultrasound in telemedicine its impact in high-risk obstetric health care delivery. Ultrasound Q 2014;30(3):167–72.
9. Nudell J, Slade A, Jovanovič L, et al. Technology and pregnancy. Int J Clin Pract Suppl 2011;65(170):55–60.
10. Tricco AC, Lillie E, Zarin W, et al. Prisma extension for scoping reviews (PRISMA-ScR): checklist and explanation. Ann Intern Med 2018;169(7):467–73.
11. United Nations Development Program. Human Development Index. Available at: http://hdr.undp.org/en/content/human-development-index-hdi. Accessed, July 10, 2019.
12. Gilliam ML, Martins SL, Bartlett E, et al. Development and testing of an iOS waiting room "app" for contraceptive counseling in a Title X family planning clinic. Am J Obstet Gynecol 2014;211:481.e1–8.
13. Smith C, Ngo TD, Gold J, et al. Effect of a mobile phone-based intervention on post-abortion contraception: a randomized controlled trial in Cambodia. Bull World Health Organ 2015;93:842–850A.
14. Chernick LS, Stockwell MS, Wu M, et al. Texting to increase contraceptive initiation among adolescents in the emergency department. J Adolesc Health 2017; 61(6):786–90.
15. Bull S, Devine S, Schmiege S, et al. Text messaging, teen outreach program, and sexual health behavior: a cluster randomized trial. Am J Public Health 2016;106:S117–24.
16. McCarthy O, Ahamed I, Kulaeva F, et al. A randomized controlled trial of an intervention delivered by mobile phone app instant messaging to increase acceptability of effective contraception among young people in Tajikistan. Reprod Health 2018;15(1):28.
17. Buchanan CRM, Tomaszewski K, Chung SE, et al. Why didn't you text me? Post-study trends from the DepoText trial. Clin Pediatr (Phila) 2018;57:82–8.
18. Castano PM, Bynum JY, Andres R, et al. Effect of daily text messages on oral contraceptive continuation: a randomized controlled trial. Obstet Gynecol 2012;119:14–20.
19. Trent M, Thompson C, Tomaszewski K. Text messaging support for urban adolescents and young adults using injectable contraception: outcomes of the DepoText pilot trial. J Adolesc Health 2015;57:100–6.
20. Hou MY, Hurwitz S, Kavanagh E, et al. Using daily text-message reminders to improve adherence with oral contraceptives: a randomized controlled trial [published erratum appears in Obstet Gynecol 2010;116:1224]. Obstet Gynecol 2010; 116:633–40.
21. Tsur L, Kozer E, Berkovitch M. The effect of drug consultation center guidance on contraceptive use among women using isotretinoin: a randomized, controlled study. J Womens Health (Larchmt) 2008;17:579–84.
22. Thiel de Bocanegra H, Bradsberry M, Lewis C, et al. Do Bedsider family planning mobile text message and e-mail reminders increase kept appointments and contraceptive coverage? Womens Health Issues 2017;27:420–5.
23. Wilkinson TA, Berardi MR, Crocker EA, et al. Feasibility of using text message reminders to increase fulfilment of emergency contraception prescriptions by adolescents [letter]. J Fam Plann Reprod Health Care 2017;43:79–80.
24. Zuniga C, Grossman D, Harrell S, et al. Breaking down barriers to birth control access: an assessment of online platforms prescribing birth control in the USA. J Telemed Telecare 2018;0(0):1–10.
25. Curtis KM, Tepper NK, Jatlaoui TC, et al. U.S. medical eligibility criteria for contraceptive use, 2016. MMWR Recomm Rep 2016;65:1–104, appendices C and D.

26. Grant R. The website providing abortion without borders. Available at: http://digg. com/2016/women-on-web. Accessed July 19 2019.
27. Aiken ARA, Digol I, Trussell J, et al. Self reported outcomes and adverse events after medical abortion through online telemedicine: population based study in the Republic of Ireland and Northern Ireland. BMJ 2017;357:j2011.
28. Gomperts R, Petow SA, Jelinska K, et al. Regional differences in surgical intervention following medical termination of pregnancy provided by telemedicine. Acta Obstet Gynecol Scand 2012;91:226–31.
29. Gomperts R, van der Vleuten K, Jelinska K, et al. Provision of medical abortion using telemedicine in Brazil. Contraception 2014;89:129–33.
30. Gomperts RJ, Jelinska K, Davies S, et al. Using telemedicine for termination of pregnancy with mifepristone and misoprostol in settings where there is no access to safe services. BJOG 2008;115:1171–5 [discussion: 5–8].
31. Les K, Gomperts R, Gemzell-Danielsson K. Experiences of women living in Hungary seeking a medical abortion online. Eur J Contracept Reprod Health Care 2017;22:360.
32. Hyland P, Raymond E, Chong E. A direct-to-patient telemedicine abortion service in Australia: retrospective analysis of the first 18 months. Aust N Z J Obstet Gynaecol 2018;58:335–40.
33. Raymond E, Chong E, Winikoff B, et al. TelAbortion: evaluation of a direct to patient telemedicine abortion service in the United States. Contraception 2019; 100(3):173–7.
34. Endler M, Beets L, Gemzell Danielsson K, et al. Safety and acceptability of medical abortion through telemedicine after 9 weeks of gestation: a population-based cohort study. BJOG 2019;126(5):609–18.
35. Wiebe ER. Use of telemedicine for providing medical abortion. Int J Gynaecol Obstet 2014;124:177.
36. Grossman D, Grindlay K. Safety of medical abortion provided through telemedicine compared with in person. Obstet Gynecol 2017;130:778–82.
37. Grossman D, Grindlay K, Buchacker T, et al. Effectiveness and acceptability of medical abortion provided through telemedicine. Obstet Gynecol 2011;118: 296–303.
38. Kohn JE, Snow JL, Simons HR, et al. Medication Abortion provided through Telemedicine in Four U.S. States. Obstet Gynecol 2019;134(2):343–50.
39. Grindlay K, Lane K, Grossman D. Women's and providers' experiences with medical abortion provided through telemedicine: a qualitative study. Womens Health Issues 2013;23:e117–22.
40. Grindlay K, Grossman D. Telemedicine provision of medical abortion in Alaska: through the provider's lens. J Telemed Telecare 2017;23:680–5.
41. Endler M, Lavelanet A, Cleeve A, et al. Telemedicine for medical abortion: a systematic review. BJOG 2019;126(9):1094–102.
42. Aiken A, Gomperts R, Trussell J. Experiences and characteristics of women seeking and completing at-home medical termination of pregnancy through online telemedicine in Ireland and Northern Ireland: a population-based analysis. BJOG 2017;124:1208–15.
43. Momberg M, Harries J, Constant D. Self-assessment of eligibility for early medical abortion using m-Health to calculate gestational age in Cape Town, South Africa: a feasibility pilot study. Reprod Health 2016;13:40.
44. Constant D, de Tolly K, Harries J, et al. Mobile phone messages to provide support to women during the home phase of medical abortion in South Africa: a randomized controlled trial. Contraception 2014;90(3):226–33.

45. de Tolly KM, Constant D. Integrating mobile phones into medical abortion provision: intervention development, use, and lessons learned from a randomized controlled trial. JMIR Mhealth Uhealth 2014;2(1):e5.
46. Guttmacher Institute. Counseling and Waiting periods for abortion. 2019. Available at: https://www.guttmacher.org/state-policy/explore/counseling-and-waiting-periods-abortion. Accessed: July 20, 2019.
47. Ehrenreich K, Kaller S, Raifman S, et al. Women's experiences using telemedicine to attend abortion information visits in Utah: a qualitative study. Womens Health Issues 2019;29(5):407–13.
48. Bracken H, Lohr PA, Taylor J, et al. RU OK? The acceptability and feasibility of remote technologies for follow-up after early medical abortion. Contraception 2014;90:29–35.
49. Ngoc N, Bracken H, Blum J, et al. Acceptability and feasibility of phone follow-up after early medical abortion in Vietnam: a randomized controlled trial. Obstet Gynecol 2014;123(1):88–95.
50. Platais I, Tsereteli T, Comendant R, et al. Acceptability and feasibility of phone follow-up with a semiquantitative urine pregnancy test after medical abortion in Moldova and Uzbekistan. Contraception 2015;91(2):178–83.
51. Chen M, Rounds K, Creinin M, et al. Comparing office and telephone follow-up after medical abortion. Contraception 2016;94:122–6.
52. Michie L, Cameron S. Simplified follow-up after early medical abortion: 12-month experience of a telephone call and self-performed low-sensitivity urine pregnancy test. Contraception 2014;84:440–5.
53. Cameron S, Glasier A, Dewart H, et al. Telephone follow-up and self-performed urine pregnancy testing after early medical abortion: a service evaluation. Contraception 2012;86:67–73.
54. McKay RJ, Rutherford L. Women's satisfaction with early home medical abortion with telephone follow-up: a questionnaire based study in the UK. J Obstet Gynaecol 2013;33(6):601–4.
55. Anger H, Dabash R, Pena M, et al. Use of an at-home multilevel pregnancy test and an automated call-in system to follow-up the outcome of medical abortion. Int J Gynaecol Obstet 2019;144:97–102.
56. Perriera LK, Reeves MF, Chen BA, et al. Feasibility of telephone follow-up after medical abortion. Contraception 2010;81:143–9.
57. Mangone ER, Lebrun V, Muessig KE. Mobile phone apps for the prevention of unintended pregnancy: a systematic review and content analysis. JMIR Mhealth Uhealth 2016;4(1):1–13.
58. Lunde B, Perry R, Sridhar A, et al. An evaluation of contraception education and health promotion applications for patients. Womens Health Issues 2017;27-1:29–35.
59. World Health Organization. Telemedicine: opportunities and developments in member states. Available at: https://www.who.int/goe/publications/goe_telemedicine_2010.pdf. Accessed July 10, 2019.
60. Center for Connected Health Policy. State telehealth laws and reimbursement Policies: a Comprehensive scan of the 50 States and the District of Columbia. Report. 2019. Available at: https://www.cchpca.org.
61. Raymond EG, Grossman D, Wiebe E, et al. Reaching women where they are: eliminating the initial in-person medical abortion visit. Contraception 2015;92(3):190–3.
62. Guttmacher Institute. Medication abortion, State Laws and Policies (as of May 2019). 2019. Available at: https://www.guttmacher.org/state-policy/explore/medication-abortion. Accessed July 20, 2019.

Connected Health and Mobile Apps in Obstetrics and Gynecology

Nathaniel DeNicola, MD, MSHP[a,b],*, Kathryn Marko, MD[a,b,c]

KEYWORDS

- Mobile application • Telemedicine • Gynecology • Obstetrics • Pregnancy
- Prenatal care • STI • Telehealth

KEY POINTS

- Telemedicine applications need to be developed with assistance from health care professionals.
- Mobile applications are increasingly popular among patients for medical purposes.
- Women's health providers should be discussing the use of mobile health apps with their patients.

INTRODUCTION

Mobile applications, or apps, are increasingly relevant in women's health. Patients and providers are utilizing apps for everything from menstrual tracking to menopause. More than 30% of cellular phone users look up health information on their device and 1 in 5 users have downloaded a health-related mobile app.[1] Among the 100,000 health-related mobile apps offered in the Apple App Store, there are more than 1800 related to obstetrics and gynecology,[2,3] yet less than 15% were considered useful to providers.[4] The technology industry is investing substantially in this sector with mobile health (mHealth) raising a record-setting $1.3 billion worldwide in 2016.[5] This significant investment has led to rapid growth and change. Medical app development also is outpacing the vetting process, and there is limited guidance as to which apps are valuable and of high quality.

[a] The George Washington University School of Medicine & Health Sciences, Washington, DC, USA; [b] The American College of Obstetricians and Gynecologists Taskforce on Telehealth, Washington, DC, USA; [c] Department of Ob/Gyn, 2150 Pennsylvania Avenue Northwest, Floor 6A, Washington, DC 20037, USA
* Corresponding author. 2150 Pennsylvania Avenue Northwest, Floor 6A, Washington, DC 20037.
E-mail address: ndenicola@gmail.com
Twitter: @NDeNicolaMD (N.D.)

Obstet Gynecol Clin N Am 47 (2020) 317–331
https://doi.org/10.1016/j.ogc.2020.02.008
0889-8545/20/© 2020 Elsevier Inc. All rights reserved.

obgyn.theclinics.com

Despite the challenges, apps can be useful tools for diagnosis, management, and education. They can bridge care gaps for the underserved. They have been shown to facilitate clinical research recruitment.[6] So how can health care providers best guide patients and themselves in this ever-changing world of digital health?

This review explores the life cycle of a digital woman using various clinical moments. In each of these moments, how provider and patient can utilize apps to improve care and experience is discussed.

CLINICAL MOMENTS
Menstrual Tracking

Clinicians encounter menstrual tracking in numerous clinical scenarios, from contraception guidance to fertility treatment, as well as symptom monitoring for abnormal uterine bleeding, such as that caused by endometriosis or polycystic ovarian syndrome. In other instances, women may track their menstrual cycles for enhanced understanding of their physical and mental states, to have supplies prepared, or to be able to accurately describe their menstrual pattern as is relates to other health care needs.[7]

For these and other varied indications, women are highly likely to use some form of personal informatics to enhance tracking of their menstrual cycle beyond the use of traditional methods, such as a paper calendar, symptom monitoring, or recall alone.[8] A recent survey found that across all age groups (<18 years old to >40 years old), 47% of women use a mobile phone app to track their menstrual cycle, and 12% use a digital calendar.[7]

Given the important clinical significance of accurate menstrual tracking and the ubiquitous use of mobile apps to enhance that recording, questions naturally follow about how this integrates into clinical practice, whether these apps provide accurate information, and if they are enhancements or risks to current standard of care.

Although data are still emerging on this topic, there are several studies to offer guidance. In terms of the educational materials that often accompany a menstrual tracking app, the data provide cause for concern. In evaluating a sample of more than 100 menstrual tracking apps, only 20% were considered clinically accurate, and few cited medical literature or health profession involvement. Furthermore, 19% of these apps contained erroneous medical information.[9]

Patient surveys do point to certain advantages for digital self-monitoring, however. Because menstruation often is treated as a personal matter, women cite the discrete nature of mobile apps as an advantage compared with keeping sensitive information on a traditional calendar. Other reported advantages of app usage include patients connecting symptoms with their menstrual cycle that otherwise had gone unnoticed, such as symptoms of depression and changes in resting heart rate. Furthermore, women state that they prefer to share this self-generated data with their health care providers.[7]

Because more than half of patients are using some form of personal informatics to track their menstrual cycle—most likely a smartphone app that can reliably record data but may be delivering inaccurate medical information—it is prudent to ask patients if they are using such an app and most importantly what they hope to achieve from it. Critical health outcomes, such as achieving or preventing pregnancy, may be linked to their intended usage, and furthermore the self-tracking might reveal new, important clinical connections, such as menstrual-related mood disruptions. Screening for—and addressing—misinformation from the apps may open opportunities for improved counseling, increased engagement, and enhanced patient experience.

Contraception

Fertility awareness–based methods

An emerging clinical aspect of digital menstrual tracking is its application to contraception, in particular, fertility awareness–based methods (FABMs). Although the integration of digital recording into traditional FABMs may seem like an obvious enhancement, it is important to not conflate technological convenience with improved clinical success. Given the critical clinical importance of an unintended pregnancy, and the heightened lay media attention to this particular form of mHealth, clinicians can expect to encounter questions regarding its utility. The current data give reasons for cautious counseling.

A study of mobile phone apps designed to avoid pregnancy found that only 6 of 30 FABM apps could predict the fertile window accurately, and the majority of apps did not incorporate evidence-based FABMs.[10] Furthermore, a systematic review of apps designed to prevent unintended pregnancy found that 41% of apps did not mention modern contraception methods, and that even when these methods were included, a majority of apps did not discuss how to use the contraceptive methods.[11] The investigators concluded that at least some of the apps in this category could increase the chance of an unintended pregnancy due to the apps' inaccuracies and lack of proper education.[11]

Perhaps more alarming are the FABM apps that specifically promote enhanced contraception success. Although there are few studies in this group, the claims warrant special attention. One industry-funded study claimed markedly improved contraception success rates by incorporating an app with FABMs, reporting a perfect-use Pearl Index of 0.5, that is, a 0.5% risk of unintended pregnancy.[12] Critically important is the finding that 7% of unplanned pregnancies for app users occurred due to the app falsely attributing a safe day within the fertile window, for example, app error that resulted in unintended pregnancies. These pregnancies were excluded from the perfect-use calculation and could provide misleading failure risks for a lay audience.

For patients who prefer FABMs, or for patients who might have a medical indication for FABM counseling (eg, contraindications for hormonal therapy), the use of apps might offer a degree of convenience and future studies eventually may demonstrate enhanced success rates. At present, however, the limited and imprecise estimates of unintended pregnancy rates using FABM apps make it premature to risk-adjust the occurrence away from the standard FABMs' pregnancy rate of 25%, and this should be included in any counseling and informed decision making.

Contraceptive education

Patient education seems a promising area of app-enhanced clinical care. In contrast to other app evaluations that raise concern, the studies thus far for contraception education generally point to user-friendly, medically accurate content that can be used by both patients and providers.[13,14] This educational material covers a range of benefits for contraception counseling and clinical efficacy.

In a study on a waiting room app, app users received educational material via a mobile device while awaiting their scheduled appointment. Not only did app users test significantly higher on knowledge of contraception effectiveness but also they reported an increased interest in long-term reversible contraception. Interactive designs and video testimonials seemed particularly effective.[15] One randomized controlled trial demonstrated that an educational mobile app could serve as an adequate and efficient adjunct to in-person contraception counseling, thus saving time for the providers.[16]

Providers also should be aware of changing legal regulations that allow a small number of remote prescribing apps for birth control pills; for example, patients obtain a prescription without an in-person physician visit. Although these remote prescribing apps remain in early development and utilization, patient satisfaction scores seem promising.

When counseling patients regarding all available contraceptive options—an increasingly wide range of options to cover—clinicians might benefit from integrating a contraception education app both to increase their clinical efficacy and to heighten patient retention of information. Similar resources exist outside of the app format in strictly Web-based platforms that may be more accessible to some populations.[17]

Fertility

Fertility and reproductive endocrinology services offer another clinical integration for women or couples interested in using a mobile app to increase their odds of conception through menstrual tracking and identification of the fertile window. Many of the app categories, discussed previously, offer dual services as fertility adjuncts. As such, much of the same precautionary counseling regarding tendencies for commercial vendors to overstate the clinical efficacy and limited accuracy in reliably identifying the fertile window still apply.

One study examined the accuracy of both Web sites and mobile apps to predict the fertile window accurately: the investigators found that although nearly all services included the most fertile cycle day, the range of the fertile window generally was inaccurate and varied widely.[18] For the provider side, a review of 2179 mobile apps intended for reproductive endocrinology and infertility providers found that only 0.32% were considered useful and that the APPLICATIONS score did not correlate with app popularity.[19]

Given the widespread popularity of menstrual tracking apps (discussed previously) and the common overlap with fertility adjuncts, clinicians should expect to encounter fertility patients who choose to integrate a mobile app into their care and be prepared to counsel on its risks and benefits. In particular, the range of inaccuracy in identifying the fertile window is important for fully informed patient utilization. Compared with apps designed to prevent pregnancy, however, the clinical effect of mislabeled fertile days for this clinical moment may be of less significance, because a majority of apps and Web sites ultimately did include the most fertile cycle day.

Pregnancy

Pregnancy is the clinical moment in which digital health technology can have the most significant impact. Women have increased engagement with health information and their provider.[20] Unfortunately, there is an unmet demand for easily accessible information in pregnancy, especially in the early part of pregnancy, when patients are seen less frequently.[21,22] Additionally, only 4% of obstetric-related Web sites were created or sponsored by a physician or midwife.[23] The remaining information available is largely inaccurate or unendorsed.[24] The challenge is to fill this void with evidence-based information.

The Text4baby program sought to do this by developing a large library of pregnancy and postpartum, evidence-based text messages.[25] These texts utilize the health belief model by sending cues for positive behavioral and attitude change while providing salient information.[26] Messaging includes information on alcohol and tobacco cessation as well as taking prenatal vitamins and seeking prenatal care. More than 700,000 women participated in the program.[27] They found the program does change attitudes and beliefs.[27,28] Regarding behaviors, in a randomized trial of 943 women using the program, they found higher levels of text message exposure predicting lower self-reported alcohol consumption postpartum (odds ratio 0.212; 95% CI, 0.046–0.973; $P = .046$).[27] This high-exposure intervention requires more study to elucidate what the appropriate dose level would be in order to have the most significant effect on behavior while avoiding information fatigue.

Not all information apps are created equal, however. In 1 study comparing free smartphone apps in pregnancy, Text4baby was found to have more content regarding postpartum planning, seeking care, and prevention and less content regarding normal pregnancy symptoms.[29] This finding demonstrates the great need and opportunity providers have to use these apps to assist in providing information to patients.

These information programs also can be used to bridge service gaps. The Text4baby program found 40% of their enrollees were from underserved zip codes (up from the 34% expected).[25] Additionally, 82% were from households where the yearly income was less than $20,000 per year.[30] Investigators also were able to identify specific barriers in this population: receipt of more than 8 text messages daily, utilizing a shared phone, and having more than 1 cell number in the past 6 months.[30] More studies need to be done to identify how these barriers can be overcome and how low health literacy affects platform utility. Internationally, the program has been adapted to the unique needs of each country. In Russia, for example, researchers found that limiting the text messages to twice weekly and providing mHealth education to providers were vital to the program's success.[31]

Information also can be provided to patients regarding test results. Although many providers utilize patient portals through their electronic health records, these portals often require a provider to authorize the results and then communicate to the patient either digitally or by mail/phone. Cheng and colleagues[32] examined patient anxiety levels while patients underwent prenatal serum screening for aneuploidy. They found that patients receiving fast result reporting by automated mobile text had mean anxiety scores less than those who had not yet received their results. The reduced anxiety, however, seemed mostly due to those with negative results. Patients with positive results had a mean anxiety score that was higher than those in the control group. Although there may be benefit to providing information quickly, these automated results do not provide the patient counseling required by some results.[32,33]

Other information apps include gestational age trackers and virtual scrapbooks. Given the pervasiveness of menstrual trackers, the unsure last menstrual period may be a thing of the past. The result is more accurate pregnancy dating and earlier care access. Virtual scrapbooks arguably are the most popular apps. Every week, patients receive an update regarding their gestational age and fetal development (eg, "Your baby is the size of an avocado!"). Although these apps are fun for the patients, they can give inaccurate or unendorsed information. Additionally, app popularity does not correlate with accuracy. These apps, however, do increase patient engagement in their pregnancies. This engagement can be transferred to partners as well. In a pilot study of a pregnancy app, 32 men whose partners were pregnant found the app useful and interesting.[34]

Unfortunately, providers can also utilize erroneous apps. Chyjeck and colleagues[3] studied 55 pregnancy wheel apps using the APPLICATIONS scoring system. They identified 55 apps and excluded 39 of these due to being consumer based, inaccurate, or both.[3]

Monitoring

Beyond information, patients and providers are seeking new ways to monitor pregnancies using mHealth technology. Outside of pregnancy, digital health tools are used to self-monitor and collect additional data points of clinical visits. In 1 study, 96 hypertensive patients were randomized to either wireless blood pressure monitoring with additional support through a mobile app and Web site or to standard care.[35] The group who received the mHealth platform had significant improvements in cigarette smoking and blood pressure control whereas the standard care group did not. In pregnancy, home blood pressure self-monitoring has been shown to be feasible and easy to use, with high patient satisfaction.[36,37] This same success has been demonstrated with blood glucose monitoring in gestational diabetes.[38] Additionally, remote glucose monitoring has been shown to decrease the hemoglobin A_{1c} of women with gestational diabetes by −0.14% (95% CI, −0.25% to −0.04%) compared with women receiving standard care.[39] Although this difference may not be clinically significant, given the improved patient satisfaction associated with mHealth initiatives and lack of demonstrable harm, similar programs likely will become more common.

Gestational weight gain is another area where mobile monitoring could have an impact. In the United States, 48% of women gain more weight than is recommended by the Institute of Medicine (IOM).[40] One intervention in women with gestational diabetes combined weight and glucose self-monitoring with automated feedback, Web-based resources, and online peer support.[41] In their cohort, 71% of participants gained within the recommended amount of weight according to IOM guidelines.

Although blood pressure, glucose, and weight are the most well-studied pregnancy monitoring tools, they are not the only ones available. Contraction monitors and kick counters also are popular. They are not necessarily accurate, however, and have no requirement for medical device vetting by the US Food and Drug Administration (FDA). Although this may not be a concern for a contraction timer, it can have serious consequences for apps that claim to be fetal heart rate monitors or Dopplers fetal heart monitors. The FDA warns that a handheld Dopplerdevices should be used only when there is a medical need and only by, or under the supervision of, a health care professional. In 2009, Chaklader and Adams[42] described a case of a nulliparous woman who felt decreased fetal movement at 38 weeks' gestation. The patient utilized a handheld Doppler devices at home, thought she heard the fetal heartbeat, and was reassured. She presented later with a fetal demise.[42] It is critical that these potential pitfalls are discussed with patients and that patients are asked if they are using these devices. Additionally, these devices cannot substitute an evaluation by a provider if concerning findings arise.

Clinical decision making

Point-of-care decision making is something obstetricians and gynecologists do on a daily basis. They have many tools at their disposal to support clinical decision making and ensure that patients are given the most accurate and up-to-date information. The Centers for Disease Control and Prevention (CDC) has many apps for both patients and providers (https://www.cdc.gov/mobile/mobileapp.html).[43] Patient apps include those on healthy eating, eating while traveling, flu, fetal alcohol spectrum disorders, and a game called "Solve the Outbreak." Providers have access to easy apps for vaccines, antibiotics, opioids, sexually transmitted disease treatment, group B streptococcus prophylaxis, and contraception.

Many societies also have sponsored apps that are well vetted, including the American College of Obstetricians and Gynecologists (ACOG), Society for Maternal-Fetal Medicine (SMFM), National Institutes of Health (NIH), and Reproductive Toxicology Center. The ACOG app has excellent guidance on immunizations, an accurate pregnancy wheel, and point-of-care access to practice bulletins and committee opinions. The Preterm Birth Toolkit and Critical Care Obstetrics are available on the SMFM app.

The NIH supports LactMed, which is a detailed description of drugs and dietary supplement use in lactation. Reprotox (Reproductive Toxicology Center) contains summaries of the reproductive effects of many drugs and chemicals with further description of the supporting evidence and citations. Some of these are stand-alone apps (CDC, SMFM, LactMed, and Reprotox) whereas others are applets, embedded within the main society apps (ACOG pregnancy wheel). Although some are free, others require society membership to access.

Remodeling care

Prenatal care is a critical to ensure healthy pregnancies and promote the best possible perinatal outcomes. The traditional 12-vist to 14-visit schedule that exists in most high-income countries, however, while providing high patient satisfaction, does not necessarily improve patient outcomes.[44] Additionally, each time a patient accesses care, there is an associated cost burden to the patient, provider, and system. Could this be an opportunity for mobile-health technology to reduce the number of prenatal visits, thereby reducing cost, yet still offer a high level of patient satisfaction?

Reduced health care costs with mHealth technology and telemonitoring already have been demonstrated in heart failure patients. Geisinger Health Plan implemented a telemonitoring program that tracked patient weight and changes in clinical condition. There was a significant reduction in hospital admission, readmission, and cost of care in the patients receiving telemonitoring.[45]

In pregnancy, there have been 2 published programs designed not only to reduce the patient visit schedule and cost but also to maintain high levels of patient satisfaction. One is OB Nest and the other is Babyscripts. OB Nest is a platform designed and implemented by the Mayo Clinic to reduce the number of prenatal visits in low-risk pregnancies while maintaining good satisfaction.[46] Patients have 8 in-office visits (with the option to have more). The platform includes remote monitoring through a home blood pressure cuff and fetal heart rate monitor. There is a dedicated nurse who is available for patient concerns and patients are connected to an online community. Results from a randomized controlled trial of 300 patients (150 in each arm) showed OB Nest provided improved satisfaction, decreased stress, and reduced number of visits (9.2 vs 11.2; $P<.0001$). There was no difference in perceived quality of care, unplanned visits, or outcomes.[47]

Babyscripts takes a similar approach, with an 8-visit schedule and home blood pressure monitoring. The platform additionally includes a wireless weight scale and mobile app.[37] The mobile app pushes a task list to patients weekly, reminding them about important upcoming tests and addressing common questions. Patients also have access to a resource list that has been vetted by their provider, filling the information gaps that exist, especially in the first trimester.[22] Patients also are asked to measure their blood pressure and weight each week. Triggers are set in place to evaluate any abnormal values via a triage algorithm that was found to have no false triggers in a pilot study.[37] With the platform, patients had increased satisfaction as well as a reduced number of visits by 43% (8.0 vs 14.0; $P<.005$).[48]

In low-resource settings, where visit frequency already is low, decreasing visits has been associated with worse perinatal outcomes.[44] mHealth technology, however, still can be helpful to improve care and access. In Madagascar, a group is using the Pregnancy and Newborn Diagnostic Assessment (PANDA).[49] The platform includes a PANDA phone and point-of-care kit that connects to a mobile unit at the hospital. The system creates an online health record that was accurate and acceptable to providers in the field. Additionally, they there were no no data lost, which is a critical component of mHealth interventions in lower-resource settings. Another area of research is in preeclampsia triage and assessment. Other investigators are examining the use of mHealth tools to assess preeclampsia risk.[50,51] The Preeclampsia Integrated Estimate of Risk On the Move is a platform utilizing a risk assessment tool and mobile phone–based pulse oximeter. The platform has been shown to be feasible and is being evaluated at a larger scale.[50] Another study is looking at the feasibility of a smartphone-based imaging and analytical tool for the Congo red dye test. This test capitalizes on the constituents in preeclamptic urine that bind the amyloidophilic dye Congo red.[51]

Ultimately, prenatal care likely will look very different in the future from what it does today, with much of that change being driven by mHealth technology.

Postpartum

Postpartum women see their providers less frequently, creating a need for information and support that could be filled with apps. Some areas that could be supported are physical activity, breastfeeding, postpartum depression screening and monitoring, and blood pressure monitoring. Postpartum women, however, may not be as engaged as are women in pregnancy or potentially are looking for different information. The effectiveness of a Facebook-delivered physical activity intervention was studied by Kernot and colleagues.[52] They found 25% of patients dropped enrollment in the postpartum period. The same decline in participation was found in the Text4baby cohort.[25] There are many breastfeeding apps available that track feedings. Additionally, the National Library of Medicine has issued LactMed, a comprehensive look at drugs and supplements in breastfeeding. A search of the app store does not reveal a significant number of apps specifically targeting postpartum depression, which may be an area where further research can be done. Given the success of home blood pressure monitoring in pregnancy, there is likely a role for home monitoring in the postpartum period.

General Gynecology

Sexually transmitted infections

Currently, apps related to sexually transmitted infections (STIs) leave something to be desired. They are an area, however, with some promise because adolescents are commonly utilizing social media and apps to discover health-related information.[53] Technologies could provide an ability to get information out to teens and racial minorities who might not have access to some programs relating to STIs. This is important particularly because more than half of all new STI infections are found in young people ages 15 to 24.[54] Currently, only approximately 15% of available apps that focus on STIs and genital infections (excluding human immunodeficiency virus [HIV]) are considered fully accurate, with 29% giving 1 or more pieces of information that were fully incorrect.[55] This poses obvious issues in the area of telehealth, because the dissemination of inaccurate information is problematic to public health.

For example, technology currently being developed to treat depression could be applied to HIV risk behaviors, providing continuous access to information, scheduling, monitoring, and awareness of locations and behaviors associated with risk behaviors.[56] Overall, these early studies show some promising applications of digital media to STI prevention and treatment.

Diet and wellness

In 2014, approximately 20% of adults owned a wearable health device, with approximately 10% wearing it daily.[57] These wearables can provide information for patients related to their overall health and their fertility as well. Apps, such as AirStrip allow for practitioners to differentiate the fetal heartbeat from the mother's both in the hospital and remotely via sensors placed on the belly, a system used by more than 3.5 million women across platforms (including the Apple Watch).[58]

A healthy diet and weight can contribute to both a healthy pregnancy, because obesity in pregnancy is associated with an increased risk of miscarriage, gestational diabetes and hypertension, and fetal macrosomia, along with an increased risk of cesarean section and shoulder dystocia.[59] Devices, such as wearable health, possibly can help with weight loss goals, because people believe that the devices help reduce obesity, and more than half of people believe that the average life expectancy will go up due to wearable health devices.[58]

Gynecologic Surgery/Inpatient

Telemedicine, when used by licensed physicians, can provide the ability to reduce admissions and conduct postoperative follow-ups without necessitating a visit to a doctor's office. Direct-to-consumer apps and Web sites raise some concerns, however, about the quality of care offered by these forms of telemedicine.[60] Also, telemedicine requires images or videos generally submitted by a patient or a staff member if a patient already is within a medical facility, with no ability for doctors to manipulate or feel the area. This sometimes can lead to a misdiagnosis where a doctor believes an issue to be far more significant than it actually is.[61]

Telemedicine, however, is being helpful in areas of surgical follow-up. One study of 96 patients found that patients were largely satisfied with a mobile phone–based telemedicine scenario, where 30 of those patients had postoperative local concerns; only 1 of those required a visit to the hospital for an in-person look at the problem.[61] Mobile app follow-up care is both suitable and cost effective for low-risk postoperative ambulatory patients, even if 1 in-person follow-up appointment is required.[62]

Menopause

Menopause can bring on several symptoms; tracking those symptoms can be beneficial to determining the best course of care. Information about symptoms can allow clinicians to better see what the problems are so as to determine treatment (hormonal vs nonhormonal, for example). There are several apps available for this purpose, 1 of which is MenoPro. MenoPro, although only available on iOS, was created in collaboration with the North American Menopause Society and provides 2 modes (1 for patients and 1 for clinicians) as well as giving access to reputable sources on menopause directly through the app.[63] Nurses also should be familiar with these apps, both for menopause and menstrual history, because the menstrual-reproductive history is a key component of women's health. Apps allow women to be more precise about the information being given, instead of relying on human recall.[64]

Urology–Gynecology

Urology also has seen an influx of apps related to the field. Apps focusing on enuresis, usually for children but useable across the board, can be found on all platforms. A 2016 study showed apps could help eliminate some of the disadvantages of pen-and-paper diaries for the evaluation of enuresis, such as poor completion rates and inconsistent patterns of entry, because most people now have access to a smartphone of some sort. The study also evaluated the available apps, with apps getting scores from 10 to 30.75 on a 50-point scale.[65] Apps that were rated lowest frequently froze or crashed, Telemedicine, via apps or other means, should be considered in the urology field. In a study of 97 unique telemedicine visits, patient satisfaction was rated very good to excellent in 95% of cases, with an average of almost 5 hours and approximately $200 saved by patients per visit.[66] As in other fields of health, however, approximately a fifth of all apps related to urology had no health care professional involvement in the development of the app and only a third were created with a scientific urology association. This is true particularly in apps targeted at the general population as opposed to targeted at clinicians.[67] Ultimately, health care professionals need to get involved in the creation of these apps for dissemination to the general public.

Gynecology–Oncology

Gynecology–oncology is an underrepresented field in the telemedicine app field. A 2016 study by Farag and colleagues[68] showed that of 748 nonconsumer gynecology–oncology apps, only 1.5% (or 11 apps) were found both useful and accurate by gynecology–oncology practitioners. The apps were found to be of varied sorts, but most were considered inaccurate or not actually related to gynecology–oncology .

Broadening the scope to oncology in general, in 2016 Kessel and colleagues[69] conducted a study evaluating health care professionals' opinions toward telemedicine and patients using medical apps; 88.9% of respondents considered telemedicine useful and nearly as many supported the idea of oncologic app, with automatic reminders, timetables, and assessments of side effects and quality of life as the most important aspects. Although there is an openness to utilizing apps in oncology, it likely will be a challenging prospect requiring stakeholders working with trustworthy institutions to create accurate apps and outcomes-based research as to the effects and benefits of such apps.[70] Some areas clinicians would like to see addressed within an app include survivorship (such as navigating the costs of cancer treatment, medication compliance, and so forth), symptom tracking, and patient engagement.

MISINFORMATION/INACCURATE INFORMATION

Throughout the authors' clinical moments, some specific areas where caution should be used when utilizing or recommending apps to patients have been identified. There are a significant number of apps that, despite their popularity, have not been vetted by medical professionals. Although this may not lead to significant harm, there are some situations, for example, smartphone-based fetal monitors, where it may. In 1 assessment of 46 apps for insulin dose calculations, 67% recommended inappropriate doses that put users at significant hypoglycemia risk or persistently suboptimal glucose control.[71] Another app purported to be able to diagnose skin cancer accurately classified only 10 of 93 biopsy-proved melanomas.[72]

Therefore, despite the appeal of mobile apps, they are not universally helpful or safe. So how can providers encourage app use that supplements care in a way that prevents patient harm? The authors encourage taking a thorough health app history. Discover what a patient is using and for what purpose. Counsel patients regarding the apps they are using and construct a clinical tool belt. Ensure the apps that are recommended have been vetted by a medical provider and use medical society-endorsed apps where possible. Finally, become a stakeholder in the industry. Partner with app developers to ensure the most accurate information is being provided to patients.

NEXT STEPS/CONCLUSIONS

Mobile apps and mHealth interventions have the potential to alter the landscape of medicine significantly, from how care is provided at the bedside to the ability to recruiting patients and conducting medical research. They have the ability to remodel prenatal care and strive toward more personalized medicine. The most remote and vulnerable patients can be reached. They must keep up with developers, however. Guidelines must be created for the optimal use of mHealth apps and a structured way to vet them. Doing this can drive the future of medicine.

DISCLOSURE

The authors have nothing to disclose.

REFERENCES

1. Smith A. U.S. smartphone use in 2015. 2015. Available at: https://www.pewresearch.org/internet/2015/04/01/us-smartphone-use-in-2015/. Accessed June 1, 2019.
2. Xu W, Liu Y. mHealthApps: a repository and database of mobile health apps. JMIR MHealth UHealth 2015;3(1):e28.
3. Chyjek K, Farag S, Chen KT. Rating pregnancy wheel applications using the APPLICATIONS scoring system. Obstet Gynecol 2015;125(6):1478–83.
4. Farag S, Chyjek K, Chen KT. Identification of iPhone and iPad applications for obstetrics and gynecology providers. Obstet Gynecol 2014;124(5):941–5.
5. Mercom Capital Group. 2016 Q4 and annual healthcare IT/digital health funding and M&A report. Available at: https://mercomcapital.com/product/2016-q4-annual-healthcare-itdigital-health-funding-ma-report/. Accessed April 20, 2017.
6. Wise LA, Rothman KJ, Mikkelsen EM, et al. Design and conduct of an internet-based. Preconception cohort study in North America: pregnancy study online. Paediatr Perinat Epidemiol 2015;29(4):360–371.e.
7. Epstein DA, Lee NB, Kang JH, et al. Examining menstrual tracking to inform the design of personal informatics tools. Proceedings of the SIGCHI Conference on Human Factors in Computing Systems. Denver, CO, May 2, 2017. doi: 10.1145/3025453.3025635.
8. Li I, Dey AK, Forlizzi J. A stage-based model of personal informatics systems. Proceedings of the SIGCHI Conference on Human Factors in Computing Systems. April 10–15, 2010. doi: 10.1145/1753326.1753409.
9. Moglia ML, Castano PM. A review of smartphone applications designed for tracking women's reproductive health. Obstet Gynecol 2015;125:41S.
10. Duane M, Contreras A, Jensen ET, et al. The performance of fertility awareness-based method apps marketed to avoid pregnancy. J Am Board Fam Med 2016; 29(4):508–11.
11. Mangone ER, Lebrun V, Muessig KE. Mobile phone apps for the prevention of unintended pregnancy: a systematic review and content analysis. JMIR MHealth UHealth 2016;4(1):e6.
12. Scherwitzl EB, Danielsson KG, Sellberg JA, et al. Fertility awareness-based mobile application for contraception. Eur J Contracept Reprod Health Care 2016; 21(3):234–41.
13. Perry R, Lunde B, Chen KT. An evaluation of contraception mobile applications for providers of family planning services. Contraception 2016;93(6):539–44.
14. Lunde B, Perry R, Sridhar A, et al. An evaluation of contraception education and health promotion applications for patients. Womens Health Issues 2017;27(1): 29–35.
15. Gilliam ML, Martins SL, Bartlett E, et al. Development and testing of an iOS waiting room "app" for contraceptive counseling in a Title X family planning clinic. Am J Obstet Gynecol 2014;211(5). https://doi.org/10.1016/j.ajog.2014.05.034.

16. Sridhar A, Chen A, Glik D. Plan a birth control: randomized controlled trial of a mobile health application. Contraception 2013;88(3):463.

17. Gawron LM, Turok DK. Pills on the World Wide Web: reducing barriers through technology. Am J Obstet Gynecol 2015;213(4). https://doi.org/10.1016/j.ajog.2015.06.002.

18. Setton R, Tierney C, Tsai T. The accuracy of web sites and cellular phone applications in predicting the fertile window. Obstet Gynecol 2016;128(1):58–63.

19. Shaia KL, Farag S, Chyjek K, et al. An evaluation of mobile applications for reproductive endocrinology and infertility providers. Telemed J E Health 2017;23(3):254–8.

20. O'Brien OA, McCarthy M, Gibney ER, et al. Technology-supported dietary and lifestyle interventions in healthy pregnant women: a systematic review. Eur J Clin Nutr 2014;68(7):760–6.

21. Grimes HA, Forster DA, Newton MS. Sources of information used by women during pregnancy to meet their information needs. Midwifery 2014;30(1). https://doi.org/10.1016/j.midw.2013.10.007.

22. Kraschnewski JL, Chuang CH, Poole ES, et al. Paging "Dr. Google": does technology fill the gap created by the prenatal care visit structure? Qualitative focus group study with pregnant women. J Med Internet Res 2014;16(6). https://doi.org/10.2196/jmir.3385.

23. Kaimal AJ, Cheng YW, Bryant AS, et al. Google obstetrics: who is educating our patients? Am J Obstet Gynecol 2008;198(6). https://doi.org/10.1016/j.ajog.2008.03.030.

24. MacNeily A. Paging Dr Google. Can Urol Assoc J 2013;7(3–4):106–7.

25. Whittaker R, Matoff-Stepp S, Meehan J, et al. Text4baby: development and implementation of a national text messaging health information service. Am J Public Health 2012;102(12):2207–13.

26. Evans WD, Abroms LC, Poropatich R, et al. Mobile health evaluation methods: the Text4baby case study. J Health Commun 2012;17(sup1):22–9.

27. Evans W, Nielsen PE, Szekely DR, et al. Dose-response effects of the Text4baby mobile health program: randomized controlled trial. JMIR Mhealth Uhealth 2015;3(1). https://doi.org/10.2196/mhealth.3909.

28. Evans WD, Wallace JL, Snider J. Pilot evaluation of the text4baby mobile health program. BMC Public Health 2012;12(1). https://doi.org/10.1186/1471-2458-12-1031.

29. Lewkowitz AK, O'Donnell BE, Nakagawa S, et al. Social media messaging in pregnancy: comparing content of Text4baby to content of free smart phone applications of pregnancy. J Matern Fetal Neonatal Med 2015;29(5):745–51.

30. Gazmararian JA, Elon L, Yang B, et al. Text4baby program: an opportunity to reach underserved pregnant and postpartum women? Matern Child Health J 2014;18(1):223–32.

31. Parker RM, Dmitrieva E, Frolov S, et al. Text4baby in the United States and Russia: an opportunity for understanding how mHealth affects maternal and child health. J Health Commun 2012;17(sup1):30–6.

32. Cheng PJ, Wu TL, Shaw SW, et al. Anxiety levels in women undergoing prenatal maternal serum screening for Down syndrome: the effect of a fast reporting system by mobile phone short-message service. Prenatal Diagn 2008;28(5):417–21.

33. Gurol-Urganci I, Jongh TD, Vodopivec-Jamsek V, et al. Mobile phone messaging for communicating results of medical investigations. Cochrane Database Syst Rev 2012. https://doi.org/10.1002/14651858.cd007456.pub2.

34. Mackert M, Guadagno M, Donovan E, et al. Including men in prenatal health: the potential of e-Health to improve birth outcomes. Telemed J E Health 2015;21(3):207–12.

35. Kim JY, Steinhubl SY, Wineinger NY. The influence of wireless self-monitoring program on the relationship between patient activation and health behaviors, medication adherence, and blood pressure levels in hypertensive patients. J Med Internet Res 2016;18(6):e116.

36. Ganapathy R, Grewal A, Castleman J. Remote monitoring of blood pressure to reduce the risk of preeclampsia related complications with an innovative use of mobile technology. Pregnancy Hypertens 2016;6(4):263–5.

37. Marko KI, Krapf JM, Meltzer AC, et al. Testing the feasibility of remote patient monitoring in prenatal care using a mobile app and connected devices: a prospective observational trial. JMIR Res Protoc 2016;5(4). https://doi.org/10.2196/resprot.6167.

38. Hirst JE, Mackillop L, Loerup L, et al. Acceptability and user satisfaction of a smartphone-based, interactive blood glucose management system in women with gestational diabetes mellitus. J Diabetes Sci Technol 2014;9(1):111–5.

39. Ming WK, Mackillop LH, Farmer AJ, et al. Telemedicine technologies for diabetes in pregnancy: a systematic review and meta-analysis. J Med Internet Res 2016;18(11). https://doi.org/10.2196/jmir.6556.

40. NVSS - Birth Data. Centers for disease control and prevention. 2019. Available at: https://www.cdc.gov/nchs/nvss/births.htm. Accessed June 1, 2019.

41. Nicholson WK, Beckham AJ, Hatley K, et al. The Gestational Diabetes Management System (GooDMomS): development, feasibility and lessons learned from a patient-informed, web-based pregnancy and postpartum lifestyle intervention. BMC Pregnancy Childbirth 2016;16(1). https://doi.org/10.1186/s12884-016-1064-z.

42. Chakladar A, Adams H. Dangers of listening to the fetal heart at home. BMJ 2009;339. https://doi.org/10.1136/bmj.b4308.

43. Mobile Apps. Centers for disease control and prevention. 2019. Available at: https://www.cdc.gov/mobile/mobileapp.html. Accessed July 19, 2019.

44. Dowswell T, Carroli G, Duley L, et al. Alternative versus standard packages of antenatal care for low-risk pregnancy. Cochrane Database Syst Rev 2015. https://doi.org/10.1002/14651858.cd000934.pub3.

45. Maeng DD, Starr AE, Tomcavage JF, et al. Can telemonitoring reduce hospitalization and cost of care? A health plans experience in managing patients with heart failure. Popul Health Manag 2014;17(6):340–4.

46. Ridgeway JL, Leblanc A, Branda M, et al. Implementation of a new prenatal care model to reduce office visits and increase connectivity and continuity of care: protocol for a mixed-methods study. BMC Pregnancy Childbirth 2015;15(1). https://doi.org/10.1186/s12884-015-0762-2.

47. Butler-Tobah YS, Leblanc A, Branda M, et al. OB nest—a novel approach to prenatal care. Obstet Gynecol 2016;127. https://doi.org/10.1097/01.aog.0000483637.05137.18.

48. Marko KI, Ganju N, Brown J, et al. Remote prenatal care monitoring with digital health tools can reduce visit frequency while improving satisfaction. Obstet Gynecol 2016;127. https://doi.org/10.1097/01.aog.0000483620.40988.df.

49. Benski AC, Stancanelli G, Scaringella S, et al. Usability and feasibility of a mobile health system to provide comprehensive antenatal care in low-income countries: PANDA mHealth pilot study in Madagascar. J Telemed Telecare 2016;23(5):536–43.

50. Lim J, Cloete G, Dunsmuir DT, et al. Usability and feasibility of PIERS on the move: an mHealth app for pre-eclampsia triage. JMIR Mhealth Uhealth 2015; 3(2). https://doi.org/10.2196/mhealth.3942.
51. Jonas SM, Deserno TM, Buhimschi CS, et al. Smartphone-based diagnostic for preeclampsia: an mHealth solution for administering the Congo Red Dot (CRD) test in settings with limited resources. J Am Med Inform Assoc 2015;23(1): 166–73.
52. Kernot J, Olds T, Lewis LK, et al. Effectiveness of a facebook-delivered physical activity intervention for post-partum women: a randomized controlled trial protocol. BMC Public Health 2013;13(1). https://doi.org/10.1186/1471-2458-13-518.
53. Gilliam ML, Chor J, Hill B. Digital media and sexually transmitted infections. Curr Opin Obstet Gynecol 2014;26(5):381–5.
54. Sexual risk behaviors can lead to HIV, STDS, & teen pregnancy. Centers for Disease Control and Prevention. 2019. Available at: https://www.cdc.gov/healthyyouth/sexualbehaviors/index.htm. Accessed July 9, 2019.
55. Gibbs J, Gkatzidou V, Tickle L, et al. 'Can you recommend any good STI apps?' A review of content, accuracy and comprehensiveness of current mobile medical applications for STIs and related genital infections. Sex Transm Infect 2016; 93(4):234–5.
56. Brown CH, Mohr DC, Gallo CG, et al. A computational future for preventing HIV in minority communities. J Acquir Immune Defic Syndr 2013;63:S72–84.
57. Health Wearables. Early days. PwC health research institute. 2014. Available at: https://www.pwc.com/us/en/health-industries/top-health-industry-issues/assets/pwc-hri-wearable-devices.pdf. Accessed November 30, 2015.
58. Tiku N. Apple watch can tell a baby's heart rate from its mom's. BuzzFeed News. 2015. Available at: https://www.buzzfeednews.com/article/nitashatiku/apple-watch-mother-baby-heartrate. Accessed November 17, 2019.
59. Moussa HN, Alrais MA, Leon MG, et al. Obesity epidemic: impact from preconception to postpartum. Future Sci OA 2016;2(3). https://doi.org/10.4155/fsoa-2016-0035.
60. Resneck JS, Abrouk M, Steuer M, et al. Choice, transparency, coordination, and quality among direct-to-consumer telemedicine websites and apps treating skin disease. JAMA Dermatol 2016;152(7):768–75.
61. Martínez-Ramos C, Cerdán MT, López RS. Mobile phone–based telemedicine system for the home follow-up of patients undergoing ambulatory surgery. Telemed J E Health 2009;15(6):531–7.
62. Armstrong KA, Semple JL, Coyte PC. Replacing ambulatory surgical follow-up visits with mobile app home monitoring: modeling cost-effective scenarios. J Med Internet Res 2014;16(9). https://doi.org/10.2196/jmir.3528.
63. MenoPro mobile App. MenoPro: a mobile app for women bothered by menopause symptoms. Available at: https://www.menopause.org/for-women/-i-menopro-i-mobile-app. Accessed November 15, 2019.
64. McCartney PR. Nursing practice with menstrual and fertility mobile apps. MCN Am J Matern Child Nurs 2016;41(1):61.
65. Myint M, Adam A, Herath S, et al. Mobile phone applications in management of enuresis: the good, the bad, and the unreliable! J Pediatr Urol 2016;12(2):e1–6.
66. Chu S, Boxer R, Madison P, et al. Veterans affairs telemedicine: bringing urologic care to remote clinics. Urology 2015;86(2):255–61.
67. Pereira-Azevedo N, Carrasquinho E, Oliveira ECD, et al. mHealth in urology: a review of experts' involvement in app development. PLoS One 2015;10(5). https://doi.org/10.1371/journal.pone.0125547.

68. Farag S, Fields J, Pereira E, et al. Identification and rating of gynecologic oncology applications using the APPLICATIONS scoring system. Obstet Gynecol 2016;22(12):1001–7.
69. Kessel KA, Vogel MM, Schmidt-Graf F, et al. Mobile apps in oncology: a survey on health care professionals' attitude toward telemedicine, mHealth, and oncological apps. J Med Internet Res 2016;18(11). https://doi.org/10.2196/jmir.6399.
70. Berkowitz CM, Zullig LL, Koontz BF, et al. Prescribing an app? Oncology providers' views on mobile health apps for cancer care. JCO Clin Cancer Inform 2017;(1):1–7.
71. Huckvale K, Adomaviciute S, Prieto JT, et al. Smartphone apps for calculating insulin dose: a systematic assessment. BMC Med 2015;13. https://doi.org/10.1186/s12916-015-0314-7.
72. Ferrero NA, Morrell DS, Burkhart CN. Skin scan: a demonstration of the need for FDA regulation of medical apps on iPhone. J Am Acad Dermatol 2013;68(3):515–6.

Telepsychiatry in Obstetrics

Linda L.M. Worley, MD[a,b,*], Alexandra Wise-Ehlers, MD[c]

KEYWORDS

- Telemedicine • Telemental health • Telepsychiatry • Postpartum depression
- Substance use in pregnancy • Maternal suicide

KEY POINTS

- Women often experience unrecognized, untreated perinatal mental illness and substance use disorders, which can have devastating effects.
- Pregnancy offers a window of opportunity for engaging a woman in treatment to improve her own health and ultimately the health and well-being of her family.
- The American College of Obstetrics and Gynecology and the American Psychiatric Association recommend routine screening, referral, and treatment of pregnant and postpartum women with these disorders.
- Access to perinatal mental health experts can be a challenge.
- Telepsychiatry provides a promising venue for connecting obstetric providers and their patients to perinatal mental health experts.

INTRODUCTION

Major depressive disorder is the leading cause of disease-related disability in women globally.[1-3] Perinatal depression affects as many as 1 in 7 women and is one of the most common complications of pregnancy and the postpartum period,[4] with potentially devastating consequences if unrecognized and untreated.[5] Other disorders, such as bipolar disorder, anxiety disorders, posttraumatic stress disorder, and substance use disorders, also negatively impact the health and well-being of women, infants, and families. Maternal suicide now exceeds hemorrhage and hypertensive disorders as a cause of maternal mortality in the first postpartum year.[5,6] Perinatal depression has been linked to lower-quality interactions between mothers and their

a Northwest Arkansas University of Arkansas for Medical Sciences (UAMS) College of Medicine, UAMS Northwest College of Medicine, UAMS, 1125 North College Avenue, Fayetteville, AR 72703, USA; b Vanderbilt, Nashville, TN, USA; c University of Arkansas for Medical Sciences, UAMS Little Rock College of Medicine, 4301 West Markham Street Slot 831, Little Rock, AR 72205, USA
* Corresponding author. Northwest Arkansas University of Arkansas for Medical Sciences (UAMS) College of Medicine, UAMS Northwest College of Medicine, UAMS, 1125 North College Avenue, Fayetteville, AR 72703.
E-mail address: WorleyLindaL@uams.edu
Twitter: @drLindaWorley (L.L.M.W.)

Obstet Gynecol Clin N Am 47 (2020) 333–340
https://doi.org/10.1016/j.ogc.2020.02.009
0889-8545/20/© 2020 Elsevier Inc. All rights reserved.
obgyn.theclinics.com

newborns,[7] higher rates of emotional and behavioral problems in the children as they grow older, worse social competence with peers, and a poorer adjustment to school overall.[8]

ILLNESSES AFFECTING THE BRAIN

Women with untreated depression, mood disorders, posttraumatic stress disorder, and anxiety disorders have a more difficult time following their obstetricians' prenatal care recommendations to discontinue cigarette, alcohol, and substance use during pregnancy.[9] The use of legally available substances, cigarettes and alcohol, is contra-indicated during pregnancy.[10] They are known teratogens that increase the risk for complications and poor outcomes (eg, small for gestational age, premature birth, neonatal withdrawal from nicotine, attention deficit disorder, sudden infant death syndrome, and mental retardation), and alcohol use in pregnancy is the most common preventable cause of mental retardation.[11] According to the National Institute on Alcohol Abuse and Alcoholism, the prevalence of fetal alcohol syndrome in the United States is 2 to 7 cases per 1000 and the prevalence of fetal alcohol spectrum disorders is as high as 20 to 50 cases per 1000.[12]

The incidence of cigarette smoking and substance use disorders is significantly associated with exposure to 4 or more adverse early childhood experiences.[13] According to the 2017 Pregnancy Risk Assessment Monitoring System (PRAMS), 17.6% of women acknowledged smoking in the 3 months before pregnancy, 8.1% in the final 3 months of pregnancy, and 11.7% in the postpartum period.[14] An estimated 33% of opioid-dependent US citizens are women of childbearing age[15] and very few (7%) inpatient treatment programs offer specialized programs for pregnant and postpartum women. Of these, slightly more than half (56%) offer the recommended medication-assisted treatment (MAT). The remaining programs (44%) only offer detoxification services, which increases the risk for relapse and poor outcomes.[16] The current American College of Obstetricians and Gynecologists' (ACOG) standard-of-care guidelines recommend MAT for pregnant women with opioid use disorders.[17]

It is common for perinatal depression to be overlooked when illness-associated changes in sleep, appetite, and libido are misattributed to the physiologic changes related to pregnancy and postpartum. Depressed women often do not disclose the depth of their suffering to their obstetricians out of fear of being judged or being seen as an unfit mother.[18] In 1 study, only 1 of every 5 women diagnosed with postpartum depression had informed her health care provider of her depressive symptoms.[5] Specific risk factors underlying maternal deaths in the postpartum year caused by suicide and opioid-related overdose are major depressive disorder, bipolar disorder, substance use disorders, and intimate partner violence.[16] The peak time for these tragic deaths is 7 to 12 months postpartum.[16]

RISK FACTORS FOR DEVELOPING PERINATAL DEPRESSION
- Personal and/or family history of depression or mood disorder[4]
- History of physical and/or sexual abuse
- Having an unplanned or unwanted pregnancy
- Current stressful life events
- Pregestational or gestational diabetes
- Complications during pregnancy (preterm delivery or pregnancy loss)
- Low socioeconomic status
- Lack of social or financial support
- Adolescent parenthood

OVERALL RECOMMENDATIONS

ACOG recommends that obstetric care providers screen patients at least once during the perinatal period for depression and anxiety symptoms using a standardized, validated tool.[1] In addition, the US Preventive Services Task Force regards this screening during the perinatal period as standard of care.[1,19] In 2018, ACOG expanded their recommendation to also completing a full assessment of mood and emotional well-being during the comprehensive postpartum visit for each patient and, when indicated, initiation of medical therapy and referral for appropriate follow-up mental health treatment.[5] For women with current depression or anxiety, a history of, and/or risks for, perinatal mood disorders (including suicidal thoughts), close monitoring, evaluation, and assessment are warranted.[5]

SCREENING TOOLS

Several screening instruments have been validated for use during pregnancy and the postpartum period to assist with systematically identifying patients with perinatal depression.[5] The Edinburgh Postnatal Depression Scale[20,21] is most frequently used. It has been translated into 50 languages, consists of 10 self-reported questions that are health literacy appropriate, and takes less than 5 minutes to complete. It also includes anxiety symptoms, which are a prominent feature of perinatal mood disorders. It excludes constitutional symptoms of depression, such as changes in sleeping patterns, energy, and appetite, which can be common in pregnancy and the postpartum period, thus making the tool more specific for identifying perinatal depression.

It is also important to screen for bipolar disorder knowing that it increases the risk for acute exacerbation in the immediate postpartum course 100-fold for the emergence of postpartum psychosis and acute mood instability.[22,23] Some providers prefer to screen by asking about past history of being able to go for days with very limited sleep while having high energy (without using drugs/illicit substances) or by using a standardized screening tool such as the Mood Disorder Questionnaire.[24,25] This tool is validated and takes approximately 5 minutes to complete.

Screening for substance use at the first prenatal visit is recommended.[17] Because of the stigmatized nature of substance use, it is important to put patients at ease using a nonjudgmental approach in the screening and intervention process. Pregnant patients with substance use disorders often have other comorbid conditions, such as posttraumatic stress disorder, depression, anxiety, and a history of abuse. It is important to be mindful of potential relapse triggers, such as loss of insurance, sleep deprivation, and caring for a newborn.

Screen for substance use early in pregnancy using a validated tool such as the national Institute on Drug Abuse (NIDA) Quick Screen.[17] If it is positive, complete the NIDA Modified ASSIST screen (adapted from the World Health Organization (WHO) Alcohol, Smoking and Substance Involvement Screening Test (ASSIST). Pregnancy offers a window of opportunity to offer hope by engaging women in treatment while their motivation is high to have a healthy pregnancy and newborn. In some states, identification and referral for substance use treatment also requires interfacing with a complex legal landscape. Obstetricians need to remain up to date with their state guidelines to do no harm. In states with punitive stances (rather than recognizing substance use disorders as medical illnesses in need of effective treatment) fear of legal ramifications and potential loss of custody deters pregnant patients from seeking prenatal care, and from honestly disclosing their struggles. Both ACOG and the American Psychiatric Association advocate for a concerted effort to retract of this type of legislation.

TREATMENT MODELS
Telepsychiatry/Telemental Health

Telepsychiatry, a use of telemedicine to provide mental health assessments and treatment at a distance, enters its sixth decade as a well-known practice,[26] with widespread adoption within the Veterans Health Administration and the armed forces. Both patients and providers report being very satisfied with its use for a wide variety of services.[27] Telemental health services use Internet-based videoconferencing technologies through personal computers and mobile devices to provide mental health and substance abuse services from a distance.[28] Mental health treatment is particularly suited to this use of advanced communication, enabling physically distant specialists to provide expert consultation and treatment of those who would not have access otherwise. Recent large randomized controlled trials have shown the effectiveness of telemental health,[28] which has been found to be effective for diagnosis and assessment across many populations in many settings.[27] In addition, new models of care (ie, collaborative care, asynchronous and mobile) have shown equally positive outcomes.[27]

Costs for telemental health are both direct and indirect, including equipment, installation of lines, and other supplies. Fixed costs include the rental cost of lines, salary and wages, and administrative expenses. Variable costs include data transmission costs, fees for service, and maintenance and upgrades of equipment.[27]

Clinical guidelines for telemental health practices[28]:

1. Verify professional and patient identity, provider's credentials and licensure information.
2. Document location of provider and patient. The professional must comply with the jurisdiction where the patient physically receives treatment. Establish appropriate emergency plan.
3. Verify contact information for professional and patient.
4. Verify expectations for contact between sessions, including a discussion of emergency management should this occur.
5. Obtain informed consent appropriate for relevant jurisdiction and document. Include discussion of structure and timing of services, record keeping, scheduling, privacy, potential risks, confidentiality in electronic communication, an agreed-on emergency plan and contact, process for patient documentation and its storage, the potential for technical failure, procedures for coordination of care with other professionals, a protocol for contact between sessions, and conditions warranting termination of telemental health services with a referral to in-person care.
6. Physical environment on both sides must be secure to ensure the privacy of the patient.
7. Plan for coordination of care with patient's treatment team.
8. Emergency management plan including the designation of a patient support person to contact in the case of an emergency.

Collaborative Model/Telepsychiatry

The collaborative model of care implemented within the obstetrician's office has good evidence for positively affecting outcomes.[29] This approach to care requires that patients undergo universal screening with evidence-based screening tools. For those with positive screens, algorithm-guided treatment is initiated by the obstetrician, who simultaneously initiates a referral to a care manager who immediately follows up with each patient, closely coordinating ongoing care and follow-up evidence-based screenings to monitor response to treatment in collaboration with the supervising, collaborating perinatal psychiatrist. The perinatal psychiatrist is available to see patients as needed either in person or via telepsychiatry, enabling high-quality care and, in some cases, across geographic distances.[29]

SUMMARY

There is broad consensus among national professional organizations that recognizing, diagnosing, and treating perinatal mental illness and substance use disorders is essential. When obstetricians screen, intervene, and refer pregnant and postpartum women in need of treatment to effective care, both mothers and babies benefit. Early universal screening for substance use followed by a brief intervention providing feedback and advice and a referral for treatment using a coordinated multidisciplinary approach (without criminal sanctions) can also improve maternal and infant outcomes.[17] Pregnancy offers an important window of opportunity to identify and engage women in treatment.[30]

Universal screening identifies more women in need of care and increases the demand for access to perinatal mental health experts. In order to meet this need, several evidence-based models of care have emerged and continue to expand across the nation. Both the collaborative model of care and the telephonic consultation service directly support obstetric providers who are responsible for initiating treatment of their patients. Telepsychiatry services go 1 step further by connecting the patient to a perinatal mental health expert who evaluates the patient over a Health Insurance Portability and Accountability Act–compliant video conferencing technology enabling face to face communication over a distance. This encounter can be a consultation service resulting in a formal evaluation, diagnosis, and treatment recommendations for the obstetrician to consider and act on, or a venue for providing ongoing perinatal mental health treatment directly to the patient.

Telemental health technologies offer great promise, but face barriers to widespread implementation:

1. Significant demand for limited numbers of perinatal mental health experts
2. Requirement for telemedicine infrastructure
3. Restricted provision of care across state lines (providers must be licensed in state where patient is receiving care)
4. Challenges in fiscal sustainability

Telepsychiatry services offer an accessible resource for obstetricians to connect patients in need of treatment to skilled perinatal mental health experts who otherwise would not have been accessible.

FUTURE DIRECTIONS

Maternal health is a growing concern garnering the attention of lawmakers and professional organizations alike. State mortality data are being closely monitored to better identify actionable causes driving unacceptable maternal mortalities. Efforts are underway to expand eligibility for access to psychiatric treatment throughout the high-risk postpartum year. Innovative models of care using telepsychiatry and emerging health technologies continue to build a strong network of collaborative partnerships between obstetricians and perinatal mental health experts across the nation.

SCREENING TOOLS

Edinburgh Postnatal Depression Scale[20,21]:
  https://www.fresno.ucsf.edu/pediatrics/downloads/edinburghscale.pdf.
  The Mood Disorder Questionnaire[24]:
  http://www.sadag.org/images/pdf/mdq.pdf.

Screening Tools from the National Institute of Drug Addiction

The NIDA Quick Screen:
  https://www.drugabuse.gov/sites/default/files/files/QuickScreen_Updated_2013(1).pdf.
  The NIDA Modified Assist Screen:
  https://www.drugabuse.gov/sites/default/files/pdf/nmassist.pdf.

RESOURCES

ACOG:
  www.acog.org/More-Info/PerinatalDepression.
  Prescription Drug Monitoring Program[17]:
  www.pdmpassist.org/content/state-profiles.
  Screening, Brief Intervention, and Referral to Treatment:
  http://www.integration.samhsas.gov/clinical-practice/SBIRT.
  State Laws:
  www.guttmacher.org/state-policy/explore/substance-abuse-during-pregnancy.
  Substance Use:
  Substance Abuse and Mental Health Administration:
  www.integration.samhsa.gov/
  https://findtreatment.samhsa.gov.

TREATMENT GUIDELINES

University of Arkansas for Medical Sciences, Department of Obstetrics and Gynecology Antenatal and Neonatal Guidelines Education and Learning System (ANGELS) obstetric guidelines:
  Anxiety (antepartum and postpartum):
  https://angelsguidelines.com/guidelines/anxiety-antepartum-and-postpartum/
  Depression (antepartum and postpartum):
  https://angelsguidelines.com/guidelines/depression-antepartum-and-postpartum/
  Domestic violence during pregnancy (intimate partner violence):
  https://angelsguidelines.com/guidelines/domestic-violence-during-pregnancy/
  Nicotine dependence:
  https://angelsguidelines.com/guidelines/nicotine-dependence/
  Opioid use disorder and other substance use during pregnancy:
  https://angelsguidelines.com/guidelines/substance-abuse-in-pregnancy/
  Psychiatric emergencies in obstetrics/acute psychiatric illness
  https://angelsguidelines.com/guidelines/psychiatric-emergencies-in-obstetricsacute-psychiatric-illness/

PERINATAL MENTAL HEALTH EXPERTS

- https://the-periscope-project.org/: The Periscope Project is a free resource for health care providers caring for pregnant and postpartum women who are struggling with mental health or substance use disorders.

- MCPAP for Moms (www.mcpapformoms.org): early implementation of telepsychiatry visits/14 perinatal psychiatry access programs across the United States in various stages of implementation, several of which will be implementing telepsychiatry.
- Lifeline4Moms (www.lifeline4moms.org).
- MySafeRx (https://www.mysaferx.org/): a mobile technology platform that integrates daily coaching and supervised medication taking to increase medication adherence, prevent overdose, and strengthen recovery. Treating postpartum women. Program is interested in expanding to treating women during pregnancy. Located at Cambridge Health Alliance in Massachusetts and Vermont.

DISCLOSURE

The authors have nothing to disclose.

REFERENCES

1. American College of Obstetricians and Gynecologists, Committee on Obstetric Practice. Committee opinion no. 453: Screening for depression during and after pregnancy. Obstet Gynecol 2010;115(2 Pt 1):394–5.
2. ACOG committee opinion no. 757. Summary: screening for perinatal depression. Obstet Gynecol 2018;132(5):1314–6.
3. Kessler RC. Epidemiology of women and depression. J Affect Disord 2003; 74(1):5–13.
4. US Preventive Services Task Force, Curry SJ, Krist AH, Owens DK, et al. Interventions to prevent perinatal depression: US preventive services task force recommendation statement. JAMA 2019;321(6):580–7.
5. ACOG committee opinion no. 757. Screening for perinatal depression. Obstet Gynecol 2018;132(5):e208–12.
6. Palladino CL, Singh V, Campbell J, et al. Homicide and suicide during the perinatal period: Findings from the national violent death reporting system. Obstet Gynecol 2011;118(5):1056–63.
7. Stein A, Gath DH, Bucher J, et al. The relationship between post-natal depression and mother-child interaction. Br J Psychiatry 1991;158:46–52.
8. Kersten-Alvarez LE, Hosman CM, Riksen-Walraven JM, et al. Early school outcomes for children of postpartum depressed mothers: comparison with a community sample. Child Psychiatry Hum Dev 2012;43(2):201–18.
9. Worley LL, Conners NA, Crone CC, et al. Building a residential treatment program for dually diagnosed women with their children. Arch Womens Ment Health 2005; 8(2):105–11.
10. ACOG. American College of Obstetricians and Gynecologists. Committee on obstetric practice: tobacco, alcohol, drugs, and pregnancy. 2019. Available at: https://www.acog.org/Patients/FAQs/Tobacco-Alcohol-Drugs-and-Pregnancy?IsMobileSet=false. Accessed November 23, 2019.
11. NIH. National institute on alcohol abuse and alcoholism: fetal alcohol exposure and the brain. Available at: https://pubs.niaaa.nih.gov/publications/aa50.htm. Accessed November 23, 2019.
12. May PA, Gossage JP, Kalberg WO, et al. Prevalence and epidemiologic characteristics of FASD from various research methods with an emphasis on recent in-school studies. Dev Disabil Res Rev 2009;15(3):176–92.
13. Merrick MT, Ford DC, Ports KA, et al. Vital signs: estimated proportion of adult health problems attributable to adverse childhood experiences and implications

for prevention - 25 states, 2015-2017. MMWR Morb Mortal Wkly Rep 2019;68(44): 999–1005.

14. CDC. Prevalence of selected maternal and child health indicators for all PRAMS sites, pregnancy risk assessment monitoring system (PRAMS), 2016-2017. Available at: https://www.cdc.gov/prams/prams-data/mch-indicators/states/pdf/selected-2016-2017-MCH-indicators-aggregate-by-site_508.pdf. Accessed November 23, 2019.

15. Unger A, Jung E, Winklbaur B, et al. Gender issues in the pharmacotherapy of opioid-addicted women: Buprenorphine. J Addict Dis 2010;29(2):217–30.

16. Mangla K, Hoffman MC, Trumpff C, et al. Maternal self-harm deaths: an unrecognized and preventable outcome. Am J Obstet Gynecol 2019;221(4):295–303.

17. Committee on Obstetric Practice. Committee opinion no. 711: opioid use and opioid use disorder in pregnancy. Obstet Gynecol 2017;130(2):e81–94.

18. Prevatt BS, Desmarais SL. Facilitators and barriers to disclosure of postpartum mood disorder symptoms to a healthcare provider. Matern Child Health J 2018; 22(1):120–9.

19. Siu AL, US Preventive Services Task Force (USPSTF), Bibbins-Domingo K, et al. Screening for depression in adults: US preventive services task force recommendation statement. JAMA 2016;315(4):380–7.

20. Cox JL, Holden JM, Sagovsky R. Detection of postnatal depression. development of the 10-item edinburgh postnatal depression scale. Br J Psychiatry 1987;150: 782–6.

21. Wisner KL, Parry BL, Piontek CM. Clinical practice. Postpartum depression. N Engl J Med 2002;347(3):194–9.

22. Heron J, McGuinness M, Blackmore ER, et al. Early postpartum symptoms in puerperal psychosis. BJOG 2008;115(3):348–53.

23. Chaudron LH, Pies RW. The relationship between postpartum psychosis and bipolar disorder: a review. J Clin Psychiatry 2003;64(11):1284–92.

24. Hirschfeld RM, Williams JB, Spitzer RL, et al. Development and validation of a screening instrument for bipolar spectrum disorder: The mood disorder questionnaire. Am J Psychiatry 2000;157(11):1873–5.

25. Clark CT, Sit DK, Driscoll K, et al. Does screening with the mdq and epds improve identification of bipolar disorder in an obstetrical sample? Depress Anxiety 2015; 32(7):518–26.

26. Hilty DM, Marks SL, Urness D, et al. Clinical and educational telepsychiatry applications: a review. Can J Psychiatry 2004;49(1):12–23.

27. Hilty DM, Ferrer DC, Parish MB, et al. The effectiveness of telemental health: a 2013 review. Telemed J E Health 2013;19(6):444–54.

28. Turvey C, Coleman M, Dennison O, et al. ATA practice guidelines for video-based online mental health services. Telemed J E Health 2013;19(9):722–30.

29. Melville JL, Reed SD, Russo J, et al. Improving care for depression in obstetrics and gynecology: a randomized controlled trial. Obstet Gynecol 2014;123(6): 1237–46.

30. McLafferty LP, Becker M, Dresner N, et al. Guidelines for the management of pregnant women with substance use disorders. Psychosomatics 2016;57(2): 115–30.

Reducing Infant Mortality Using Telemedicine and Implementation Science

Clare Nesmith, MD[a], Franscesca Miquel-Verges, MD[b],
Tara Venable, MD[a], Laura E. Carr, MD[a], Richard W. Hall, MD[a],*

KEYWORDS

- Telemedicine • Perinatal regionalization • Infant mortality • Implementation science
- Infant • Premature

KEY POINTS

- Perinatal regionalization is an evidence-based strategy to lower infant mortality.
- Barriers to perinatal regionalization can be mitigated using implementation science.
- Telemedicine is a critical tool for the implementation of an optimal perinatal regionalization strategy.
- Telemedicine can be used effectively to engage and educate community providers and stakeholders aiming to lower infant mortality.
- Telemedicine can be used to support appropriate referral and back transport of preterm and sick neonates

INTRODUCTION

Perinatal regionalization is an evidence-based strategy to reduce infant mortality (IM). The inability to implement optimal perinatal regionalization results in preventable infant deaths for very low birthweight (VLBW, <1500 g) infants.[1,2] Perinatal regionalization is achieved by establishing systems designating where neonates are born according to the level of care needed, regardless of financial need, race, or ethnicity. Regionalized systems assign hospitals risk-appropriate levels, and ensure high-risk neonates are born in facilities with appropriate technology and specialized health care providers, such as maternal fetal medicine and neonatology specialists.[3] Nationally, health care payment systems and institutional prestige have led to a trend toward

[a] Division of Neonatology, Department of Pediatrics, University of Arkansas for Medical Sciences, Slot 512 B, 4301 West Markham, Little Rock, AR 72205, USA; [b] 1 Children's Way Slot 512-5, Little Rock, AR 72202, USA
* Corresponding author.
E-mail address: hallrichardw@uams.edu

Obstet Gynecol Clin N Am 47 (2020) 341–352
https://doi.org/10.1016/j.ogc.2020.02.010
0889-8545/20/© 2020 Elsevier Inc. All rights reserved.

deregionalization, resulting in higher IM.[4] *This trend, which is under provider control, results in the deaths of thousands of neonates every year in the United States, and minorities share the burden disproportionately.* The United States lags behind 28 other industrialized nations in IM, and there are significant disparities in this country, in large part because of failure to implement optimal regionalization.[5] Implementation strategies consist of engaging stakeholders (providers, payers, parents, and advocates) as champions, harnessing telemedicine connectivity, and using academic rigor to implement optimal regionalization.

BENEFITS OF PERINATAL REGIONALIZATION

The American College of Obstetricians and Gynecologists (ACOG) and the American Academy of Pediatrics (AAP) classify levels of care into levels 1 to 4, with AAP and ACOG level 1 providing basic care and level 4 providing the most sophisticated care. The emphasis from regionalization advocates has been on the AAP levels of care guidelines, but in February 2015, ACOG published a consensus guideline for maternal levels of care that generally correspond to the AAP levels. Research demonstrates VLBW neonatal mortality is lower for infants born at level 3 or 4 centers compared with those born in non–level 3 centers. In addition, evidence also shows IM of VLBW neonates is much higher at low-volume neonatal intensive care units (NICUs). The relative risk of death in NICUs with fewer than 25 VLBW annual admissions is 2.2 compared with high-volume NICUs with more than 100 annual VLBW admissions.[6] However, not all studies have found a significant effect of volume on IM. Rogowski and colleagues[7] found that NICU volume contributed only 9% to the variance in IM mortality using data from the large Vermont-Oxford network. However, the Vermont-Oxford Network database, while including mortality as a data point, also includes transfer to another facility. Thus, if a neonatal patient is transferred to another higher-level facility (for example, to a children's hospital for surgical treatment of necrotizing enterocolitis), then dies, the death may not be recorded as a death in the transferring hospital's database. Using Department of Health data, volume in Arkansas was found to be a significant contributor to IM (**Fig. 1**). Clearly, local data for each state or region should be used to determine specific requirements for designating level of care.

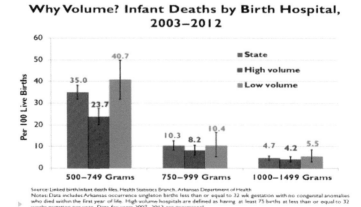

Fig. 1. Differences in infant mortality in Arkansas in low (<50 annual VLBW deliveries) versus high (>100 VLBW annual deliveries).

Intraventricular hemorrhage (IVH) causes significant adverse neuro-developmental sequelae for premature newborns.[8] IVH, as well as other morbidities associated with prematurity are lower when infants are delivered in a higher level of care hospital. Numerous studies have demonstrated that if infants are delivered where they are cared for after delivery, their risk for an IVH is less.[9,10] It is unclear whether the increased IVH rate is due to the transport itself or the difference in care at hospitals with lower levels of care. Regardless, to prevent adverse neurodevelopmental outcome, there is a significant benefit to delivering high-risk pregnancies in an appropriate-level hospital where their care can be continued until discharge or stable for back transport.

BARRIERS TO OPTIMAL REGIONALIZATION

Multiple barriers to regionalization exist. Regionalization requires complicated coordination and consensus among providers, hospitals, and patients.[11] In a study of adult clinicians and administrators in a variety of hospital settings, multiple barriers were identified. Barriers include those that affect the patient and the patient's family, the clinicians, and the hospitals. Traveling to a regional center puts an emotional and financial burden on the patient and family, particularly if the hospitalization is prolonged. One study found clinicians identified a loss of autonomy and income as barriers to regionalization and were concerned that reaching agreement among providers would be unlikely.[12] Further, regionalization has financial consequences for both the referring hospital as well as the accepting regional center. The same study also identified lack of a strong central authority and regulation in the area of regionalization as additional barriers.[12] In a subsequent national survey, adult intensivists proposed solutions to barriers to regionalization of care. These included the development of common information technology platforms across hospitals, using objective criteria to determine need for transfer, providing financial incentives to the referring hospitals and clinicians, and demonstrating through a clinical trial the benefits of regionalization.[13]

Similar barriers are found in regionalization of perinatal care. However, in the care of the mother and newborn, the coordination becomes more complicated and the burden to the family can be higher if the mother-newborn dyad is separated. Prestige and revenue are key barriers to transferring infants to hospitals with appropriate levels of care. The mean NICU charge for a baby weighing less than 1000 g at the Arkansas Perinatal Center was $124,171 in 2016 (Hall RW, 2016,unpublished data). Thus, transferring even one small neonate out of a smaller community hospital can seriously affect the referring hospital's financial viability. Further, in Arkansas, as in many other states, transferring a mother will cause the obstetric provider to lose 90% of the patient charge. Prestige is affected because some hospitals, providers, and patients interpret transferring patients as an indicator of poor performance of the community hospital, even though transferring to a higher level of care is a sign of best practice. Thus, even though data supporting regionalization of neonatal care are compelling, implementing that practice is challenging. **Table 1** summarizes barriers to perinatal regionalization and how they were addressed in Arkansas.

TELEMEDICINE HAS BEEN USED SUCCESSFULLY TO FACILITATE COOPERATION AMONG RURAL PROVIDERS

The benefits of telemedicine are highlighted when evaluating its ability to effect change in rural communities. These communities are important to the success of optimal perinatal regionalization because they are often classified at a lower level and low volume so they have to transfer infants out to achieve optimal neonatal

Table 1
Barriers to regionalization of neonatal care and methods of overcoming them

Barriers	Specific Issue	How Barriers Were Addressed
Loss of income	Loss of income for the referring provider and hospital	Back transport once patient stable Minimize patients needing referral out based on Arkansas infant mortality data Adopt slogan of "best care closest to home"
Loss of prestige	Perception of referral out meant inadequate local care	Data from Arkansas Department of Health shows improved outcome with appropriate referral Education of providers Peer pressure to "do the right thing"
Initial cost of telemedicine equipment	$162,000 (Telemedicine investment)	Initial funding from grant (National Institutes of Health) and local philanthropy Sustainable hospital investment over time because of ability to use the technology long term Infrastructure cost and support staff frequently estimated at $5000 annually
Connectivity	Inadequate bandwidth	Adequate bandwidth has become the norm in community hospitals
Community provider time	Local provider time for census rounds	Nurses participated in tele-nursery rounds (10 min 3 times wkly); physician participation needed only when specific questions or issues were raised
Perinatal provider time	Perinatal center provider time	Time needed was 1 h weekly Goodwill and enhanced communication made up for the slight drain on academic time
Lack of education	Education for community providers needed	Peds PLACE: wkly educational conferences connecting the perinatal center with community practices; community providers had input into lecture topics; free continuing medical education credits were offered

care. According to the US Census Bureau, as of December 2016, approximately 19.3% of the population live in rural areas, the equivalent of approximately 60 million people.[14] In Arkansas, approximately 42% of residents live in a rural county.[15] Rural communities have been well-labeled as health disparity populations, defined by the National Institutes of Health as a population in which there is "a significant disparity in the overall rate of disease incidence, prevalence, morbidity, or mortality in the specified population as compared with the general population."[16] These patients often have difficulty obtaining access to care as a result of the uneven distribution and relative shortage of medical care providers, issues that have persisted despite considerable efforts by both federal and state governments to address these health disparities.[17] As a result, rural patients find themselves with higher rates of disease and increased mortality, underscoring the need for easier, more readily available access to care, which can be addressed through the use of telemedicine. In fact, when implemented, telemedicine has proven to be valuable in facilitating cooperation among rural providers and specialists to decrease mortality and morbidity among certain patient populations. Developed by Dr Arora, Project ECHO (Extension for Community Healthcare Outcomes) demonstrated that the use of videoconferencing was successful in treating chronic hepatitis C infection in underserved, rural communities. His study compared treatment of patients at the University of New Mexico hepatitis C clinic with those treated by their primary care clinicians at specified ECHO clinic sites in rural areas and prisons in New Mexico. The primary endpoint was sustained virologic response, with the study showing that a total of 57.5% of patients treated at the University of New Mexico hepatitis C clinic and 58.2% of those treated at the ECHO sites had a sustained viral response.[18] These results are encouraging, revealing that when videoconferencing is used by rural providers to cooperate with specialists in the care of patients, telemedicine then becomes an effective way to treat disease in underserved communities. Telemedicine has similarly proven its value in rural communities, as demonstrated by Portnoy and colleagues[19] comparing asthma control between children seen at an in-person visit and those seen at a telemedicine session at a local, rural clinic using real-time equipment and a telefacilitator. A total of 34 in-person and 40 telemedicine patients completed all 3 visits, including an initial visit, a follow-up visit at 30 d, and a follow-up visit at 6 months. The results showed that all had a small, although statistically insignificant, improvement in their asthma control over time, and, most importantly, revealed that telemedicine was not inferior to in-person visits. It is not difficult, then, to see the many advantages that telemedicine can afford rural communities, particularly its ability to confer coordination of care among rural providers with specialists not readily available in-person. This coordination of care among rural providers via telemedicine has shown itself to be a promising vehicle for changing the landscape of disparate health care and related morbidity and mortality in rural America. Successful use of telemedicine is a key player in reducing IM by allowing for optimal perinatal regionalization and cooperation among rural health care providers and their urban specialists.

USE OF TELEMEDICINE IN OBSTETRICS

The ANGELS (Antenatal and Neonatal Guidelines, Education and Learning System) program has demonstrated how telemedicine can improve health care in a rural state like Arkansas. Telemedicine in Arkansas has allowed obstetricians to provide subspecialty care to rural areas for families with limited resources and has improved access to high-risk obstetrics for these families. In rural states such as Arkansas with remote areas, a high-risk center, through the use of telemedicine, can provide patients with the expertise of maternal fetal medicine specialists and geneticists. Through the use of teleultrasound technology, Health Insurance Portability and Accountability Act (HIPAA)-compliant broadband connections, and high-definition video, subspecialty expertise becomes available for complicated pregnancies in rural communities. For example, Fisk and colleagues[20] found that teleultrasound resulted in significantly fewer referrals to a specialist compared with those who did not have teleultrasound.

Because telemedicine provides real-time secure medical care, a plan for complicated pregnancies may be formulated allowing the family to ask questions and actively participate in the plan of care without traveling long distances. Barriers to subspecialty care, such as transportation, child care, time off work, and travel expenses, are addressed through consultation via telemedicine. Through virtually uniting patients, their local providers, and subspecialists, one study found changes to the management plan for 45.8% of the cases when a subspecialist comanaged via telemedicine with the generalist over management by a generalist alone. Patient satisfaction and the patient-physician relationship was not compromised, as 95% of the pregnant women in the study would highly recommend videoconferencing to others.1. Magann EF, Bronstein J, McKelvey SS, Wendel P, Smith DM, Lowery CL. Evolving trends in maternal fetal medicine referrals in a rural state using telemedicine. Archives of Gynecology & Obstetrics 2012;286:1383-92.

Using telemedicine, subspecialists can provide real-time interpretation of images and guide ultrasounds in rural areas. Through subspecialist-guided teleultrasound, the patient and generalist have access to real-time diagnosis and planning for delivery. Fetal diagnosis of congenital heart disease by telemedicine was found by McCrossan, and colleagues[21] to be 97% accurate. This accuracy affords communities with limited access to health care the advantage of subspecialists working with generalists to provide quality care. Arkansas used the existing educational interactive video network, then equipped rural hospitals with telemedicine equipment and broadband. This allowed a system used for education to also provide an avenue for consultation with specialists, genetic counselors, and ultrasounds available through the academic medical center. As these diagnoses are identified, a specific plan of care can be formulated by the family, the generalist, and the subspecialist to provide the best maternal and neonatal outcomes.

TECHNICAL REQUIREMENTS FOR TELEMEDICINE USE IN PERINATAL REGIONALIZATION

Generally, synchronous or live telemedicine is needed for this purpose because real-time interaction is needed for videoconferencing as well as neonatal assessment.[22] Sufficient audio-video quality is needed for appropriate patient assessment and provider communication. For example, an adequate assessment of respiratory distress in a neonate will require equipment capable of displaying respiratory effort, degree of nasal flaring, and degree of costal retractions. A single photo in time does not adequately portray respiratory effort in a neonate. Equipment required varies from software-based systems to turn-key videoconferencing units. Peripheral medical devices may be needed depending on the type of telemedicine being practiced. These devices can be hardwired or portable and include a stethoscope, otoscope, ophthalmoscope, pulse ox, or electrocardiogram.[23]

The American Telemedicine Association recommends a minimum of 640 × 360-pixel resolution at 30 frames per second transmission for video cameras. However, this is low definition, and the practical minimum standard should be high-definition video, with 1920 × 1080-pixel resolution recommended. The technology should support H.264 video compression standard or better, H.261 video compression compatibility, and G.711 audio compression standard or better to provide high-quality video and audio interaction.[22] Telemedicine also requires adequate bandwidth, as most use a high-speed Internet connection. A connectivity speed of 384 kbps for standard video and 1 mbps for high-definition video is recommended.[23] All technologies need to comply with legal, organizational, and regulatory requirements that will likely change as more technology develops.

Year-round information technology (IT) support is an essential part of telemedicine connectivity. Having someone available to ensure connectivity requires infrastructure capable of responding when there are technical issues. The IT personnel must be well trained in the equipment and be able to troubleshoot problems that may arise in the middle of the night.

TELEMEDICINE WAS USED EXTENSIVELY TO IMPLEMENT REGIONALIZATION OF NEONATAL INTENSIVE CARE IN ARKANSAS

In 2005, Arkansas was 1 of only 3 states in the United States without a formal system of perinatal regionalization. After evaluation of Arkansas Department of Health IM data linking delivery hospital to IM, the Arkansas Department of Health formed a Perinatal Advisory Committee to address the problem and provide solutions with the goal of lowering IM through perinatal regionalization[24] (**Fig. 2**). Telemedicine was used to provide clinical care and education in the following ways[2]:

- 24 hour/7 day obstetric consultation through telemedicine.
- 24 hour/7 day neonatal consultation through telemedicine.
- Weekly educational conference (Peds PLACE) emphasizing interaction with community providers.
- Telemedicine "census rounds" 3 times per week involving community hospital providers and the academic center to assess appropriate back transport candidates, and provide follow-up on those patients referred to higher level of care.
- Obstetric census rounds twice weekly to assess need for transport to a higher level of care.

Arkansas was successful in implementing regionalized NICU care, changing the pattern of neonatal deliveries in telemedicine-equipped hospitals, which resulted in significantly lower IM.[2] Formative evaluations were used throughout the implementation process of regionalization. The formative evaluation process began with a granular assessment of IM data related to birthing hospital. The Arkansas Department of Health provided unbiased rigorous statistical assessment to evaluate the statewide hospital data. The implementation strategies used in Arkansas were centered around monthly 90-minute stakeholder meetings. Stakeholders included academic and

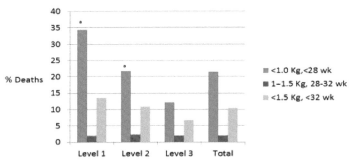

Fig. 2. IM in designated nursery levels in Arkansas, 2001–2007. [a] *P*<.001. (Source: Arkansas Department of Health.)

community providers (physicians and/or hospital administrators) from *all* level 3 hospitals, the Arkansas Department of Health, Arkansas Hospital Association, March of Dimes, Arkansas Medicaid, Arkansas Chapter of the AAP, and parent representatives. Other strategies included a physician champion, telemedicine to engage rural community providers, technical assistance, and education (Peds PLACE). The Children's Hospital CEO, who was perceived to be authoritative and unbiased, chaired the committee. Formative evaluation and these implementation strategies have been used successfully in other contexts to improve guideline adoption.[25,26] The process was organized conceptually around the 4 stages of the Simpson Transfer Model, which has been used in a variety of technology adaptations. Its use in Arkansas and how telemedicine was used to implement those strategies are described in **Table 2**.[27] The model was successful as judged by the increase in the maternal transfer of mothers expected to deliver VLBW neonates to appropriate hospitals (**Fig. 3**). Data on IM were supplied by the Arkansas Department of Health. Without telemedicine, the committee would not have been able to engage the community partners on a regular basis, as they were all at least 2 hours' driving distance from the Perinatal Advisory meeting place. Community hospital stakeholder input throughout the process was essential for buy-in, especially because the hospitals and providers were being asked to give up patients (and revenue) to the larger perinatal centers. In addition, participation of all stakeholders throughout the process gave them the opportunity to review the data showing improved IM for the smallest infants at the larger perinatal centers. Peer pressure may have played a role in the ultimate acceptance of the perinatal guidelines. Finally, the community hospitals asked and received data on IM and hospital of delivery as they requested it. Ultimately, the process proved successful statewide, with a significant reduction in IM (**Fig. 4**). In conclusion, telemedicine allowed the community hospitals and providers to participate fully in the process of regionalization without having to leave their own institution, saving time and money.

HOW CAN IMPLEMENTATION SCIENCE, USING TELEMEDICINE, BE USED IN OTHER STATES?

Widespread implementation of perinatal regionalization has not been achieved in many states, despite efforts by multiple groups such as respected national organizations and state health departments.[28] *Implementation science is the study of methods*

Table 2		
Utilization of Simpson transfer model		
Stage	**Methods**	**How Telemedicine Was Used**
Exposure	Committee formed and exposed to the infant mortality (IM) data and place of delivery of very low birthweight neonates	Community neonatologists, pediatricians connected via telemedicine
Adoption	Intention to try a new approach to implementation of regionalization of care	Robust discussion over telemedicine by 2 groups adamantly opposed to outside control
Implementation	Exploratory evaluation of IM data, effects on census	Connectivity to the Department of Health, potential use in back transport
Practice	Frequent discussions over effects of regionalization	Frequent discussions regarding back transport candidates, clinical issues

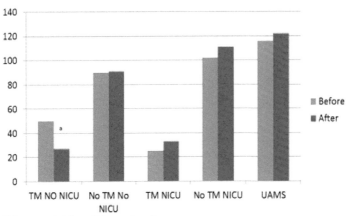

Change in number of deliveries before and after telemedicine intervention

TM represents telemedicine equipped nursery

Fig. 3. Differences in VLBW deliveries before versus after intervention in telemedicine-equipped hospitals. [a] $P = .0099$. Other values not significant.

and strategies to promote the uptake of interventions that have proven effective into routine practice, with the aim of improving population health. Using telemedicine technology, it was used to address the problem of perinatal regionalization. Although national guidelines provide an essential framework, implementation of optimal perinatal regionalization requires state-specific data. State and community-based support are essential for broad adoption of perinatal regionalization. Because states and communities have different cultures, ethnic groups, and laws, a "one-size-fits-all" approach is impractical. Although the literature is clear on the benefits of regionalization, there is little guidance on how to implement it. In Arkansas, telemedicine was used to initiate conversations with providers and stakeholders from rural communities regarding

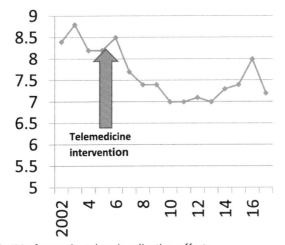

Fig. 4. Change in IM after perinatal regionalization efforts.

Table 3	
Strategies to optimize perinatal regionalization and lower infant mortality	
Process	**Specific Requirements**
Form stakeholder committee	Representatives from *all* community hospitals caring for very low birthweight neonates, American Academy of Pediatrics, American College of Obstetricians and Gynecologists, Medical Society, Hospital Association, March of Dimes, Health Department, academic institution, parent(s), administrative assistance.
Chair	Authoritative, unbiased.
Champion	Authoritative, unbiased (may or may not be the chair).
Telemedicine	*Connect all stakeholders, especially those in community hospitals. Local adaptation, understanding, and buy-in are essential.*
Technical assistance	Ability to troubleshoot telemedicine and connectivity issues.
Data acquisition	Reliable, unbiased. Granular assessment of data relating hospital of birth to infant mortality. Health Department data are ideal. Consider eliminating congenital anomalies, infants weighing less than 400 g.
Formative evaluation	Begin with granular data assessment, *focus* on infant mortality, process is data driven, encourage discussion of barriers from families, hospital chief executive officers, care providers, and families. Discuss how many infants can be saved; discuss effects of regionalization on all stakeholders; discuss various payment models; discuss quality indicators, such as volume.
Pilot testing	Test strategies to change delivery patterns, change in infant mortality.
Adapt strategies	Change strategies based on success or failure of pilot testing, assess fidelity to strategies.
Adopt strategies	Adopt successful strategies statewide, assess fidelity.

regionalization of care. The Arkansas implementation strategy package consisted of frequent telemedicine contacts (3 times weekly) with obstetric and pediatric providers in level 2 nurseries, a weekly pediatric educational conference with an emphasis on regionalization of care but with offerings related to other common pediatric problems, and 24/7 telemedicine consultation by maternal fetal medicine and neonatology providers at the perinatal center. The same strategy can be used by other states with telemedical connectivity.

Data provided by the Arkansas Department of Health were critical to the education of providers in Arkansas. Health department data can be used in other states because it is state-specific and trusted,. Thus, reliable evidence is essential to support regionalization of care in any state. The most difficult hurdle was that smaller rural nurseries would have to give up some of their patients to the larger nurseries. Telemedicine helped to overcome that obstacle by disseminating the Department of Health data, providing education to all stakeholders, including hospital administrators, payers, nurses, and physicians. An aggressive back transport program, returning infants back to the referring hospital once they were stable, was seen as supporting local hospitals. Finally, trust was enhanced by the frequent contact. A suggested format for implementation strategies to optimize perinatal regionalization is summarized in **Table 3**.

SUMMARY

Perinatal regionalization is an effective way to lower IM. Despite the known advantages of perinatal regionalization, multiple barriers exist to its implementation. Implementation science, using telemedicine, can be used to overcome those barriers, enhancing the relationship between large perinatal centers and community hospitals.

DISCLOSURE

COBRE grant, NIGMS P20 103425.

REFERENCES

1. Lorch SA, Baiocchi M, Ahlberg CE, et al. The differential impact of delivery hospital on the outcomes of premature infants. Pediatrics 2012;130:270–8.
2. Kim EW, Teague-Ross TJ, Greenfield WW, et al. Telemedicine collaboration improves perinatal regionalization and lowers statewide infant mortality. J Perinatol 2013;33:725–30.
3. Hall-Barrow J, Hall RW, Burke BL Jr. Telemedicine and neonatal regionalization of care - ensuring that the right baby gets to the right nursery. Pediatr Ann 2009;38: 557–61.
4. Wall SN, Handler AS, Park CG. Hospital factors and nontransfer of small babies: a marker of deregionalized perinatal care? J Perinatology 2004;24:351–9.
5. Available at: www.cia.gov/library/publications/the-world-factbook/rankorder/2091rank.html.
6. Phibbs CS, Baker LC, Caughey AB, et al. Level and volume of neonatal intensive care and mortality in very-low-birth-weight infants. N Engl J Med 2007;356: 2165–75.
7. Rogowski JA, Horbar JD, Staiger DO, et al. Indirect vs direct hospital quality indicators for very low-birth-weight infants. JAMA 2004;291:202–9.
8. Bassan H, Limperopoulos C, Visconti K, et al. Neurodevelopmental outcome in survivors of periventricular hemorrhagic infarction. [see comment]. Pediatrics 2007;120:785–92.
9. Palmer KG, Kronsberg SS, Barton BA, et al. Effect of inborn versus outborn delivery on clinical outcomes in ventilated preterm neonates: secondary results from the NEOPAIN trial. J Perinatology 2005;25:270–5.
10. Towers CV, Bonebrake R, Padilla G, et al. The effect of transport on the rate of severe intraventricular hemorrhage in very low birth weight infants. Obstet Gynecol 2000;95:291–5.
11. Taylor JS, Shew SB. Impact of societal factors and health care delivery systems on gastroschisis outcomes. Semin Pediatr Surg 2018;27:316–20.
12. Kahn JM, Asch RJ, Iwashyna TJ, et al. Perceived barriers to the regionalization of adult critical care in the United States: a qualitative preliminary study. BMC Health Serv Res 2008;8:239.
13. Kahn JM, Asch RJ, Iwashyna TJ, et al. Physician attitudes toward regionalization of adult critical care: a national survey. Crit Care Med 2009;37:2149–54.
14. 2010 Census Urban and Rural Classification and Urban Area Criteria. 2010. Available at: https://www.census.gov/geo/reference/ua/urban-rural-2010.html.
15. Cartwright RD. Rural profile of Arkansas. University of Arkansas System Division of Agriculture; 2017. Available at: https://www.uaex.edu/publications/pdf/MP541.pdf.

16. Minority health and health disparities research and education act United States Public Law 106-525. Available at: https://www.govinfo.gov/content/pkg/PLAW-106publ525/pdf/PLAW-106publ525.pdf. 2000. p. 2498.
17. Hart LG, Salsberg E, Phillips DM, et al. Rural health care providers in the United States. J Rural Health 2002;18(Suppl):211–32.
18. Arora S, Thornton K, Murata G, et al. Outcomes of treatment for hepatitis C virus infection by primary care providers. N Engl J Med 2011;364:2199–207.
19. Portnoy JM, Waller M, De Lurgio S, et al. Telemedicine is as effective as in-person visits for patients with asthma. Ann Allergy Asthma Immunol 2016;117:241–5.
20. Fisk NM, Sepulveda W, Drysdale K, et al. Fetal telemedicine: six month pilot of real-time ultrasound and video consultation between the Isle of Wight and London. Br J Obstet Gynaecol 1996;103:1092–5.
21. McCrossan BA, Sands AJ, Kileen T, et al. Fetal diagnosis of congenital heart disease by telemedicine. Arch Dis Child Fetal Neonatal Ed 2011;96:F394–7.
22. Burke BL Jr, Hall RW, Section On Telehealth Care. Telemedicine: pediatric applications. Pediatrics 2015;136:e293–308.
23. Marcin JP. Telemedicine in the pediatric intensive care unit. Pediatr Clin North Am 2013;60:581–92.
24. Nugent R, Golden WE, Hall R, et al. Locations and outcomes of premature births in Arkansas. J Ark Med Soc 2011;107:258–9.
25. Naik AD, Lawrence B, Kiefer L, et al. Building a primary care/research partnership: lessons learned from a telehealth intervention for diabetes and depression. Fam Pract 2015;32:216–23.
26. Freed J, Lowe C, Flodgren G, et al. Telemedicine: Is it really worth it? A perspective from evidence and experience. J Innov Health Inform 2018;25:14–8.
27. Simpson DD. A conceptual framework for transferring research to practice. J Subst Abuse Treat 2002;22:171–82.
28. Kastenberg ZJ, Lee HC, Profit J, et al. Effect of deregionalized care on mortality in very low-birth-weight infants with necrotizing enterocolitis. JAMA Pediatr 2015; 169:26–32.

Telemedicine and Distance Learning for Obstetrician/ Gynecologist Provider Education

Barbara L. Smith, RN, BSN[a],*, Lindsey B. Sward, MD[b],
Stanley K. Ellis, EdD[c]

KEYWORDS

- Tele-education • Videoconference • Teleconference • Telementoring
- Distance learning • Distance health • Digital health

KEY POINTS

- Distance learning via tele-education is a viable option for educating and disseminating best practices to rural and urban providers.
- At the University of Arkansas for Medical Sciences (UAMS), tele-education has been used in the education of OB/GYN providers for more than two decades.
- Tele-education at UAMS is interdisciplinary, using a variety of teleconferences and digital platforms.
- Tele-education will continue to advance as health care and technology evolve.

INTRODUCTION

Telemedicine is the use of "electronic…and communications technologies to provide and support healthcare when distance separates the participants."[1] Tele-education, then, is the subset of telemedicine using these technologies to support health care providers. In tele-education, communications technologies are used to distribute knowledge from one health care provider to another when distance separates the providers,[2] thus the term "distance learning." Tele-education can take many forms, but the primary goal is providing education from an urban or academic hospital (the hub) to a more rural facility (the spoke).[3]

Videoconferencing, also known as interactive video, is perhaps the most recognized form of tele-education, allowing engagement between off-site participants and on-site speakers and leading experts.[3,4] With interactive videoconferencing, which is often

[a] UAMS High-Risk Pregnancy Program, University of Arkansas for Medical Sciences, 4301 West Markham Street, Slot 519-1, Little Rock, AR 72205, USA; [b] Department of Obstetrics & Gynecology, University of Arkansas for Medical Sciences, 4301 West Markham Street, Slot 518, Little Rock, AR 72205, USA; [c] University of Arkansas for Medical Sciences, Institute for Digital Health & Innovation, 4301 West Markham Street, Slot 519, Little Rock, AR 72205, USA
* Corresponding author.
E-mail address: SmithBarbaraL@uams.edu

Obstet Gynecol Clin N Am 47 (2020) 353–362
https://doi.org/10.1016/j.ogc.2020.02.005
0889-8545/20/© 2020 Elsevier Inc. All rights reserved.

obgyn.theclinics.com

case-based,[4] off-site learners are engaged in a task and in interaction with peers. This type of education is more effective compared with more passive forms, such as distribution of information.[5] Videoconferencing has been shown to increase physician knowledge[6] and allows rural physicians to improve their knowledge without traveling long distances and without lost productivity, a common by-product of travel.[3,6]

Other forms of tele-education exist. Examples of these forms are online modules and formal and informal telementoring. Online modules allow for asynchronous learning that is interactive but is accessed at the convenience of the learner.[3,7] Formal telementoring used experts from a hub facility to guide less-experienced rural practitioners in the management of more complex disease processes.[8,9] An example telementoring effort is Project ECHO (Extension for Community Healthcare Outcomes), based at the University of New Mexico Health Sciences Center in Albuquerque.[10] Project ECHO offers a unique approach to continuing medical education by pairing clinicians with specialists at academic medical centers. This is done through teleconferencing, giving clinicians access to education on how to treat complex, chronic conditions.[10] Although it is not necessarily labeled as telementoring, informal education and mentoring occur each time a more rural provider sees a patient in a telemedicine consultation with experts who are located at an academic institution. As the separated providers work through the patient's management, knowledge about that particular patient and disease process is transferred from one provider to the other, although it may not be a formal educational event.

Significant health care disparities exist between rural and urban populations in the United States. Use of distance learning or tele-education to expand the knowledge of spoke practitioners aids in providing equitable access to quality care and evidence-based practice.[11] Arkansas, with a population of 3 million, is a rural and impoverished state with known resulting health care disparities. Recent census data show that more than one-third of the state's population lives in rural areas and, of the people living in rural Arkansas, about 20% live in poverty.[12] Of Arkansas' 75 counties, 59 are on the United States Health Resources & Services Administration's list of medically underserved areas, areas where residents have a shortage of personal health services or a lack of access to primary care.[13] Residents of rural Arkansas tend to have poorer health behaviors, access to quality care, and health outcomes in relation to Arkansans who live in urban areas.[12]

Physicians who practice in rural Arkansas, like all rural physicians in the nation, do so in geographic isolation and often with limited access to professional development.[6] Tele-education provides continuing education (CE), a means of reducing isolation, and meaningful interactions with peers without the disadvantage of required travel. Because distance health networks reduce isolation, they have been shown to have a positive effect on the recruitment and retention of providers to rural areas.[11] Tele-education, with its impact on the training and retention of rural providers, is an effective weapon in the battle against health care inequity in rural areas[3,11] and has been used in Arkansas for many years.

BACKGROUND

More than 20 years ago, a novel interactive video conference began as a collegial exchange between obstetric physicians practicing in rural areas of Arkansas and maternal-fetal medicine specialists located centrally at the state's academic medical center, the University of Arkansas for Medical Sciences (UAMS). Diverging from the traditional didactic, knowledge-focused continuing medical education program, the conference innovators invited health care providers in rural areas to participate in weekly discussions about obstetric practices with maternal-fetal medicine specialists. Participants were encouraged to ask questions, raise concerns, and provide case studies that were pertinent to the week's discussion. This interaction allowed rural and urban providers to discuss realistic approaches for best practices in their diverse clinical settings. The teleconference provided the convenience of distance learning and built relationships among obstetric colleagues based on mutual learning experiences and collaboration.

This education and support for rural providers served as a cornerstone for the development of a comprehensive program created to correct health care disparities and improve obstetric and neonatal health care statewide. In 2003, with funding through the Arkansas Medicaid program and support from the Arkansas State Medical Society, UAMS launched a multifaceted obstetric telemedicine program, the Antenatal and Neonatal Guidelines, Education, and Learning System (ANGELS). The program was designed to improve high-risk pregnancy outcomes by addressing the shortage of specialty obstetric care in rural Arkansas.[14] The ANGELS program used telemedicine networks to facilitate referrals and consultations to maternal-fetal medicine specialists for rural patients. ANGELS also provided continuing medical education to practitioners around the state.[15]

In 2003, using an already-existing interactive video network, ANGELS equipped community hospitals, free of charge, with telemedicine equipment and broadband connectivity to offer telemedicine services and CE. To facilitate the delivery of telemedicine services, a leader was identified at each spoke site who supported the new comanagement of patients by obstetric specialists at UAMS. The program began with six distant sites and was a working partnership between the maternal-fetal medicine specialists at UAMS and the medical providers throughout the state, providing information and access to the specialty services needed to ensure the success of high-risk pregnancies. The innovative use of telemedicine provided expansive support and CE for local obstetricians and family medicine practitioners in rural areas of the state.[14]

In addition to providing distance learning statewide, ANGELS offered its high-risk obstetrics teleconference to neighboring states and internationally in collaboration with obstetric providers and other health care providers at hospitals and universities in Russia, India, Ecuador, and Germany. Based on the success of the initial obstetric teleconferences and using similar methodology, additional interactive video conferences soon followed, including cross-organizational and multidisciplinary discussions to improve prenatal and postnatal genetic care, weekly teleconferences devoted to obstetric and neonatal nursing, and weekly forums for pediatric providers. Leveraging these teleconferencing capacities, other educational programs once only available at the academic medical center were easily transmitted to learners across the region.

Beginning in 2003, more than 150 obstetric and neonatal guidelines were developed and made freely accessible from a computer or mobile device at https:// angelsguidelines.com. Tailored for Arkansas' women and infants, the guidelines combined national evidence-based standards with clinical experience plus offered information about resources available in Arkansas. The guidelines were developed as a collaborative effort that included more than 200 expert Arkansan authors and reviewers from multiple disciplines and out-of-state physician peer reviewers. The intent of the guidelines was to promote best practices for health care delivery in Arkansas based on scientific evidence, national standards, and expert consensus.[16]

Throughout the history of the ANGELS program, the state's areas of greatest need were the focus for services and education. The Mississippi Delta Region, one of the most distressed areas in the nation, challenged health care providers with a population faced with stark disparities, poor accessibility to care amid rampant poverty, and low educational attainment among a rural, medically underserved population.

To help meet this challenge, ANGELS launched an innovative project to develop distance learning curricula specifically to address topics relevant to maternal-child health leadership, competencies, and evidence-based practice in the Delta. The program began in 2010 with invited participants originating from a range of disciplines with the common denominator being a desire to learn about maternal-child health topics and the racial, ethnic, and cultural health care themes within the Delta. Two interactive video conferences served as the beginning for the educational offerings: obstetrics and gynecology (OB/GYN) grand rounds and ONE Team (obstetric, neonatal, and pediatric nursing exchange), held weekly to discuss best practices in maternal-child nursing.

Included with this project was the development and implementation of an online professional learning management system that provided live streaming, content modules, and other World Wide Web–based educational materials for health care providers. The provider education portal (LearnOnDemand.org) allowed health care providers to obtain CE credit for completing online modules and professional education activities at their own pace at any time.[17]

From the beginning, ANGELS offered educational opportunities on request from outside sites, such as nursing review courses, fetal monitoring courses, and neonatal resuscitation instruction. In September 2009, casual requests for education became urgent in response to the outbreak of a novel strain of influenza sweeping the state.

As a rapid response to the severe illnesses among pregnant women and infants in the 2009 outbreak of H1N1 influenza, vital information was communicated effectively and in a timely fashion to existing telemedicine and teleconference sites across Arkansas. Health care providers acquired the latest information in an efficient manner. ANGELS responded to this demand by joining together urban and rural health care providers through interactive video teleconferences. These teleconferences served as a problem-solving forum among various disciplines and included physician experts from infectious disease, obstetrics, maternal-fetal medicine, pediatrics, neonatology, family medicine, and emergency medicine. Nursing specialists, infection control practitioners, and Arkansas Department of Health experts contributed to the discussions. More than 85 sites registered to attend the teleconferences, and health care providers unable to attend via interactive video were able to participate online via streaming video. This real-time educational response to the severe illnesses among pregnant women and infants in the outbreak of H1N1 influenza maximized the educational value of a successful statewide videoconferencing system and demonstrated the quality of service possible.[18]

Five years later, when the Ebola virus was first identified in a patient in the United States, education about Ebola and procedures for its identification and control needed immediate dissemination to health care providers. Because a state neighboring Arkansas had a diagnosed patient with the virus, many health care providers were calling to speak with public health authorities and infectious disease specialists. Additionally, the public and providers needed to be reassured that a process was in place to manage Ebola should it arrive in Arkansas.

With experience and continued growth of the network following the first rapid educational response for the H1N1 outbreak, the state's telemedicine network was prepared. In October 2014, UAMS partnered with the Arkansas Department of Health to use the UAMS Center for Distance Health's interactive video network using telehealth equipment at more than 400 sites in Arkansas. This partnership allowed the state's medical leadership to manage concerns over a potential Ebola epidemic. Six events were conducted over 4 days. Eighty-two individual health care facilities (67 of which were hospitals) used 144 individual interactive video units to connect via interactive video. A total of 378 individuals, including health care providers and the lay public, attended via webinar, and 323 health care professionals received CE credit. The existing telehealth network and infrastructure, along with established partnerships, made a rapid response possible.[19]

By 2013, the network included multiple partners and agencies and reached 454 sites. It offered access to a range of services rarely found in rural areas. Medical provider "champions" were instrumental in supporting the network, improving its infrastructure, and expanding the network into new medical disciplines and specialties. Although the network's primary function was to deliver interactive video medical consultations that united patients, local providers, and distant specialists, the network was key to delivering high-quality provider education. The telemedicine programs were accompanied by related provider-based educational efforts that fostered camaraderie between specialists and rural providers. It was also found that patients whose providers participated in ANGELS educational teleconferences were also more likely to participate in telemedicine consultation.[14]

In the years following, adequate bandwidth continued to be essential, but dedicated network connectivity no longer was a necessity. By 2018, this shift in technology allowed access to the program's education without dedicated circuits. This growth in technology allowed access from any smart device with connectivity in Arkansas that had a camera, microphone, and a screen. The advances in cellular technology and increased broadband access has greatly expanded the reach of this technology.

CURRENT EDUCATIONAL ANGELS CONFERENCES AND OTHER RESOURCES
Conferences

Each of the following conferences is aptly designated a regularly scheduled series because of their regular and recurring schedule. Through the UAMS Office of Continuing Education, CE credits are offered for each of these events. Additionally, those who are unable to connect to the conferences synchronously are afforded the opportunity to view many of the same teleconferences via the interactive Learn On Demand (LOD) learning management system.

High-risk obstetrics teleconference
The high-risk obstetrics teleconference, the flagship interactive videoconference, is still in existence today. The focus of this live teleconference is the opportunity for obstetrics providers in remote locations to discuss patient management and best practices with maternal-fetal medicine specialists. Maternal-fetal medicine specialists lead this collaborative forum that allows participants to review evidence-based practices in high-risk obstetrics using a case-based format. The previously mentioned ANGELS Obstetric and Neonatal Guidelines serve as an online resource of best practices that are often discussed during the teleconferences.

Obstetrics and gynecology grand rounds
The UAMS Department of Obstetrics and Gynecology hosts the OB/GYN Grand Rounds teleconference. The grand rounds provide physicians and other medical professionals the opportunity to present clinical and research topics relating to major women's health concerns. Physicians throughout the state are invited to listen in, participate, and ask questions of the presenters and content experts.

Obstetric and neonatal exchange team

ONE Team is a nurse-centric teleconference offered more than 20 times per year. During this teleconference, nurses are engaged in discussions of obstetric, neonatal, women's health, and pediatric issues that relate to the everyday practice of their discipline. Of particular focus during this teleconference is the use of evidence-based practice and current standards for patient care by nursing professionals.

PedsPlace

Using a telemedicine conference format, UAMS, in a collaborative effort with Arkansas Children's Hospital, addresses a single and different problem facing pediatric patients. This conference is held on a weekly schedule with the Children's Hospital as the host site. PedsPlace is facilitated on an interactive platform to engage participants in discussions that are assembled around a pediatric problem.

Connecting across professions

This multidisciplinary teleconference focuses on chronic disease, health care trends, professional development, and interprofessional collaboration. This teleconference is designed for and in partnership with Regional Programs faculty. The UAMS Regional Programs is an educational and clinical outreach network that encourages medical and other health professions graduates to remain in Arkansas. Additionally, this outreach network helps address the state's shortage and uneven distribution of primary care physicians.[20]

Lactation symposium

In conjunction with the Arkansas Breastfeeding Coalition, the ANGELS education team has coordinated an annual lactation symposium since 2012, the only lactation conference of its type offered in the state. Attendees include nurses, certified lactation consultants, dieticians, and paraprofessional peer counselors who provide breastfeeding support through the Arkansas Women, Infants & Children Program. In addition to the interactive video teleconferences, computer-based modules have been developed for provider and patient breastfeeding education.

Resources

Learn On Demand

LOD was born as a new and innovative technology that would improve evidence-based educational opportunities in maternal child health for rural health care providers in the Mississippi Delta Region.[17] The LearnOnDemand.org World Wide Web portal offers health care professionals the flexibility of earning CE credits on their schedule via an expanded array of teleconferences and online courses. The first educational modules available on LOD were videotaped lectures of departmental teleconferences (OB-GYN Grand Rounds, ONE Team, and Connecting Across Professions). As the Web site evolved, other entities began to distribute their online education content through the LOD World Wide Web portal. LOD also functions to track all educational hours and credits earned inside or outside the program and ensures compliance with the CE requirements of the national accrediting organizations for physicians and nurses. LOD users can also earn certificates of attendance for a variety of other health care disciplines.

As a testament to the demand for flexible distance learning, by 2018 usage of the Web site had grown to more than 12,000 users, encompassing 45 states, 38 countries, and 35 professions. In that year alone, the educational Web site issued more than 76,000 CE credits and hosted more than 1000 activities composed of weekly teleconferences, enduring materials, and live conferences.

Patients Learn
In 2014, Patients Learn (PatientsLearn.org) was developed to educate patients and provide them the most up-to-date medical information in an easily accessible and user-friendly format. Patients Learn serves as a robust patient resource and includes a vast knowledge-base that has been gleaned from health care providers, educators, and researchers with the intent of improving health outcomes in the state. Patients Learn includes content in the form of:

a. Interactive and engaging online courses that inform patients on myriad health and wellness issues
b. Short videos covering information on more than 100 medications
c. Informational videos that focus on specific health issues (ie, breastfeeding, childbirth, diabetes, stroke prevention, cancer, surgery care, mental health)

ANGELS guidelines
The ANGELS Obstetric and Neonatal Guidelines serve as a repository of best practice guidelines for clinicians around the state of Arkansas. The guidelines offer essential, easily accessible, and well-organized clinical information and serve as references for practicing physicians and advanced health care providers. The guidelines continue to be annually reviewed and updated by content experts and have now been converted into a mobile-friendly platform. They serve as a quick guide and local resource in an easy-to-navigate, readily available format through the angelsguidelines.com World Wide Web portal.

RESIDENT AND STUDENT EDUCATION

Although our teleconferences focus on tele-education in the context of CE for providers and professionals, tele-education is also applied in the training of undergraduate and graduate medical learners nationally and internationally.[21] At UAMS, countless medical students and residents have been a part of telemedicine and tele-education programs. Residents from various fields (including OB/GYN, pediatrics, and family medicine) and medical students participate in many of the aforementioned tele-education videoconferences at the UAMS and Arkansas Children's Hospital hub sites and at spoke sites across the state. Students and residents are also encouraged to engage with the ANGELS Obstetric and Neonatal Guidelines, using them as references for their studies.

Residents and medical students also have the opportunity to engage in telemedicine visits between patients and providers as members of the patient care team. In this way, they benefit from informal telementoring. Through these clinical encounters, residents and medical students are privy to the passage of medical knowledge from hub site provider to spoke site provider and from provider to patient. As they watch and participate in the work-up of the patient, they learn how to care for numerous high-risk and chronic conditions. Aside from medical knowledge, they also have the opportunity to learn about telemedicine as a form of care delivery. There is much to learn about this system of patient care, including technical skills, interprofessional teamwork, and the art of delivering care through telemedicine.[22]

Tele-education is also used in a more formal way in medical student education at UAMS. Students doing clinical rotations at a satellite campus in the Northwest part of Arkansas are connected to didactic sessions taught by educators at the main UAMS campus in Central Arkansas at the convenience of both parties. This has allowed remote learners to have access to the same clinical experts as students at the hub campus. Remote students are able to discuss with the lecturer in real-time and be a part of learning activities with students at the main academic facility. In this way, medical students at all UAMS locations have the opportunity to experience equal access to educational events.

THE FUTURE OF TELE-EDUCATION

As telecommunications technology becomes more widely available, cost-effective, and advanced, tele-education will continue to evolve. More advanced applications of tele-education are already on the horizon, such as surgical telementoring. In this combined form of telemedicine and telementoring, a surgeon in one location guides another, less experienced surgeon in a remote location through an operation. Thus, a patient receives advanced surgical care that he or she may previously have had to travel miles from home to receive.[23]

Another innovation in tele-education is telesimulation, in which experts at a hub facility use telecommunication technology to run simulations for management of emergent situations at a spoke facility. For instance, interactive video communications technology has been used in simulated resuscitation of adult and neonatal patients.[24–26] In the same vein, telesimulation could be used to run simulations on obstetric emergencies, such as the management of eclampsia and postpartum hemorrhage. The goal of telesimulation would ultimately be to use interactive video technology in real-time to facilitate patient care in actual resuscitation and emergency situations in spoke facilities. This type of technology has been used in the care of acute stroke[27] and could be adapted to obstetric and neonatal emergencies.

One of the greatest needs in telehealth in the future is adequate training. As telemedicine and tele-education become more ingrained in the health care system, formal educational curricula will be needed for all parties involved. Providers from various health care sectors will require more deliberate training in the telehealth delivery of patient care and provider education. Core competencies in telehealth, as developed by accrediting bodies, should be included in academic programs that provide medical education.[22]

Additional peer-review publications documenting the methodologies, successes, and lessons learned of tele-education programs throughout the nation are needed to create a more robust, comprehensive review of what is developing in OB/GYN tele-education.

SUMMARY

Tele-education uses telecommunications technology to disseminate knowledge and best practices between providers separated by distance. For more than two decades, UAMS has offered patient and provider consultations, education and training, and other services through the telehealth program. As a result, the ANGELS program has been hailed as a technological trailblazer in the world of health care delivery and health care education and training. ANGELS served as a model to be replicated in other UAMS health care disciplines. What began as a few videoconferences more than 20 years ago has evolved into a wide variety of educational programs for provider and patient education using tele-education and digital technology as platforms.

DISCLOSURE

The authors have nothing to disclose.

REFERENCES

1. Institute of Medicine.Telemedicine: a guide to assessing telecommunications for health care. Washington, DC: The National Academies Press; 1996.
2. Chiswell M, Smissen A, Ugalde A, et al. Using webinars for the education of health professionals and people affected by cancer: processes and evaluation. J Cancer Educ 2018;33(3):583–91.
3. Zollo SA, Kienzle MG, Henshaw Z, et al. Tele-education in a telemedicine environment: implications for rural health care and academic medical centers. J Med Syst 1999;23(2):107–22.
4. Regueiro MD, Greer JB, Binion DG, et al. The inflammatory bowel disease live interinstitutional and interdisciplinary videoconference education (IBD LIVE) series. Inflamm Bowel Dis 2014;20(10):1687–95.
5. Topaz M, Rao A, Masterson Creber R, et al. Educating clinicians on new elements incorporated into the electronic health record: theories, evidence, and one educational project. Comput Inform Nurs 2013;31(8):375–9 [quiz: 380–1].
6. McWilliams T, Hendricks J, Twigg D, et al. Burns education for non-burn specialist clinicians in western Australia. Burns 2015;41(2):301–7.
7. Greiner AL. Telemedicine applications in obstetrics and gynecology. Clin Obstet Gynecol 2017;60(4):853–66.
8. Arora S, Kalishman S, Thornton K, et al. Expanding access to hepatitis C virus treatment–extension for community healthcare outcomes (ECHO) project: disruptive innovation in specialty care. Hepatology 2010;52(3):1124–33.
9. Cofta-Woerpel L, Lam C, Reitzel LR, et al. A tele-mentoring tobacco cessation case consultation and education model for healthcare providers in community mental health centers. Cogent Med 2018;5(1). https://doi.org/10.1080/2331205X.2018.1430652.
10. Zigmond J. Teaching by telementoring. project ECHO advancing physicians' skill sets. Mod Healthc 2013;43(37):28–9, 35.
11. Bagayoko CO, Gagnon MP, Traore D, et al. E-health, another mechanism to recruit and retain healthcare professionals in remote areas: lessons learned from EQUI-ResHuS project in Mali. BMC Med Inform Decis Mak 2014;14:120.
12. Miller W, Knapp T. Rural Profile of Arkansas. 2019. Available at https://www.uaex.edu/publications/pdf/MP551.pdf.
13. Health Resources & Services Administration. Available at: https://www.hrsa.gov/. Accessed May 6, 2019.
14. Lowery CL, Bronstein JM, Benton TL, et al. Distributing medical expertise: the evolution and impact of telemedicine in Arkansas. Health Aff (Millwood) 2014; 33(2):235–43.
15. ACOG committee opinion no. 586: Health disparities in rural women. Obstet Gynecol 2014;123(2 Pt 1):384–8.
16. Smith BL. Evidence-based guidelines. ANGELS Annual Report 2017-2018. 2018:10-11. Available at: https://angels.uams.edu/wp-content/uploads/sites/81/2019/02/2018-Angels-annual-report-1901383a.pdf.
17. Rhoads S, Smith B. Delta interactive solution to collaborate over video for education and resources for maternal child health. J Obstet Gynecol Neonatal Nurs 2012;41(S1):S60.
18. Smith BL. ANGELS responds to H1N1 concerns. The ANGELS Report. 2009(Fall). Quarterly Newsletter published by the University of Arkansas for Medical Sciences.

19. Rhoads SJ, Bush E, Haselow D, et al. Mobilizing a statewide network to provide Ebola education and support. Telemed J E Health 2016;22(2):153–8.
20. History of Regional Programs. UAMS Regional Programs Annual Report 2017-2018. 2018:2. Available at: https://regionalprograms.uams.edu/wpcontent/uploads/sites/128/2019/10/2018_REP.pdf.
21. Lamba P. Teleconferencing in medical education: a useful tool. Australas Med J 2011;4(8):442–7.
22. Hollander JE, Davis TM, Doarn C, et al. Recommendations from the first national academic consortium of telehealth. Popul Health Manag 2018;21(4):271–7.
23. El-Sabawi B, Magee W 3rd. The evolution of surgical telementoring: current applications and future directions. Ann Transl Med 2016;4(20):391.
24. Fang JL, Carey WA, Lang TR, et al. Real-time video communication improves provider performance in a simulated neonatal resuscitation. Resuscitation 2014;85(11):1518–22.
25. Donaldson RI, Mulligan DA, Nugent K, et al. Using tele-education to train civilian physicians in an area of active conflict: certifying Iraqi physicians in pediatric advanced life support from the united states. J Pediatr 2011;159(3):507–9.e1.
26. Skorning M, Bergrath S, Rortgen D, et al. Teleconsultation in pre-hospital emergency medical services: real-time telemedical support in a prospective controlled simulation study. Resuscitation 2012;83(5):626–32.
27. Richard S, Mione G, Varoqui C, et al. Simulation training for emergency teams to manage acute ischemic stroke by telemedicine. Medicine (Baltimore) 2016;95(24):e3924.

Moving?

Make sure your subscription moves with you!

To notify us of your new address, find your **Clinics Account Number** (located on your mailing label above your name), and contact customer service at:

Email: journalscustomerservice-usa@elsevier.com

800-654-2452 (subscribers in the U.S. & Canada)
314-447-8871 (subscribers outside of the U.S. & Canada)

Fax number: 314-447-8029

Elsevier Health Sciences Division
Subscription Customer Service
3251 Riverport Lane
Maryland Heights, MO 63043

*To ensure uninterrupted delivery of your subscription, please notify us at least 4 weeks in advance of move.

Printed and bound by CPI Group (UK) Ltd, Croydon, CR0 4YY

03/10/2024

01040477-0010